# Contents

# Credits

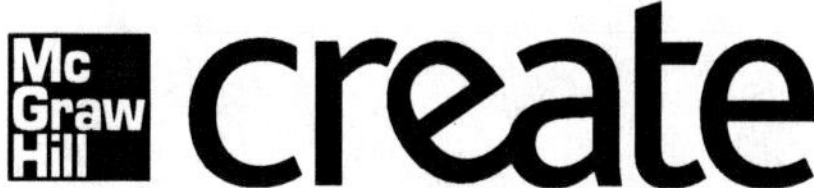

| Course | Medical Office Handbook |
| --- | --- |
| Course Number | **HS 100** |
| | **Printed For** |
| | The Allied Health Institute |
| | **ARCHITECTURE** |

The McGraw-Hill Companies

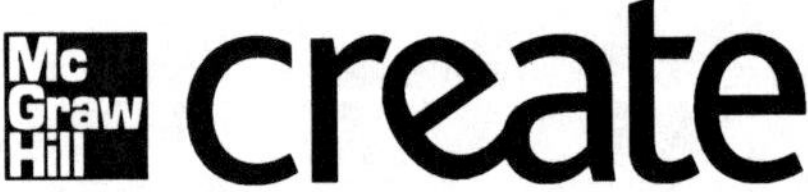


http://create.mcgraw-hill.com



ISBN-10: 1121242847 ISBN-13: 9781121242845

# Preface

The *Complete Medical Office Handbook* is a handy resource for both students on their internship or going to their first job and the seasoned professional who has been in the medical office for years. The medical office is a busy place with many day-to-day challenges. Each chapter of the *Handbook* was written to provide readers with a practical summary of the critical information they need to know. Sample forms, checklists and letters, as well as resources for more information are included.

The *Handbook* is organized into four sections.

- Part 1 covers a variety of communication topics. Chapter 1 is about the first impressions your practice makes when the patient first arrives. Chapter 2 covers general communication skills, and Chapter 3 provides a review of basic writing principles.
- Part 2 provides the reader with a primer in computer applications (Chapter 4) as well as a chapter on the various ways to schedule appointments (Chapter 5).
- Part 3 is all about the paperwork. We all know there is too much paperwork, but having a fundamental understanding of medical terminology (Chapter 6), medical records and privacy (Chapter 7), health insurance (Chapter 8), basing medical coding (Chapter 9), and the daily management of accounts (Chapter 10) is important in the day-to-day management of the medical practice.
- The last section covers safety and wellness. Safety (Chapter 11) is no longer just infection control and OSHA standards, but is also preparing for that catastrophic event—whether caused by weather or by man—all medical practices need to prepare for the unthinkable. To end the *Handbook,* a chapter on stress management will help you to better deal with the challenges in the busy office environment.

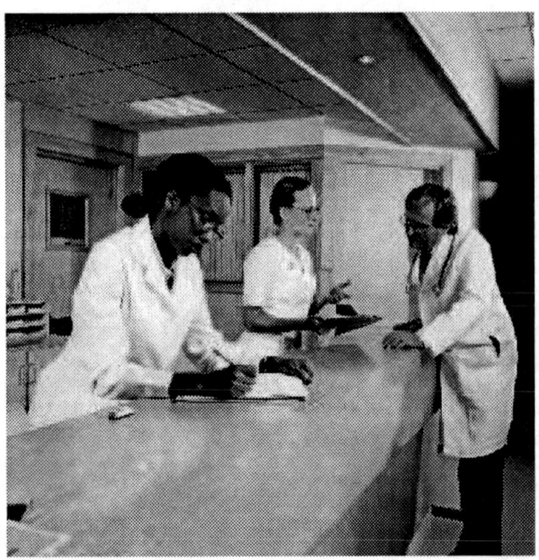

The *Complete Medical Office Handbook* is designed to be a well-used reference for the medical office staff. It is also a reference tool for the allied health student first starting out in the fastest-growing industry in the country. Working in the medical office provides us with great opportunities and challenges. This book will help you meet some of those challenges.

# Features

## Introduction

Each chapter starts with a brief introduction that gives a description about the chapter's topic, how it fits into the medical office, and why it is important for the student to be knowledgeable on the subject.

**Introduction** *In any business, records must be kept. In the medical office, the medical record or chart is the most important record that is kept. The medical record serves a variety of purposes for the practice. The importance of an accurate medical record cannot be overstated. All medical records are considered private, and maintaining that privacy is critical for all staff members to keep in mind.*

## Chapter Outline

A chapter outline provides a quick page reference for the reader to look up a topic or an important form at a glance.

*Chapter Outline*



## Summary

At the end of each chapter, a summary provides a recap of important information and reminders for the reader.

**Summary**

Learning medical terminology is important for your success in the medical office. You are probably already familiar with many medical terms. Be sure you learn the meaning of those terms that are specific to your office. Remember that many medical terms are made up of interchangeable word parts that are used in different combinations to form the word. Also remember that there may be more than one word that means the same thing. Become comfortable with the words so that you have a better understanding of what is happening in your office.

# Communications

# Part 1

## Communications

# Chapter 1

# First Impressions

## Introduction

*The medical office is a place of business. As such, the first place patients see is the reception area. The first person patients see is the receptionist. Both make a lasting impression. Maintaining a positive environment for patients while they wait to see a physician or other health care provider is important. The environment is not just the reception area itself, but the professional appearance of the staff.*

Chapter Outline



## Reception Area Basics

The look and feel of the medical office reception area is an important way to ensure the patients' comfort level. The physical environment can make patients and their families or friends feel uncomfortable and sometimes even intimidated. Let's look at both the **tangibles** and **intangibles** when it comes to the reception area.

### The Tangibles

Is the reception area clean? Would you feel comfortable if you were a patient or a member of the patient's family? Are there appropriate reading materials available? Are the walls and the fabric on the furniture done in calming colors? Is the furniture arranged properly? Is the room at a moderate temperature? Is the lighting appropriate? Do patients have privacy when checking in? Is the area free from clutter? Are educational materials available? Is the reception area safe from hazards that could cause injuries? Does the entire office provide an environment friendly to individuals who are disabled? To determine if the reception area is a comfortable place to wait in, you should assess the tangibles.

**Cleanliness and Comfort.** Medical offices usually have a cleaning company clean the offices every evening. However, since the reception area has so many people in it throughout the day, it is important to check the area periodically during the day. Watch for spills and clean them up immediately. During the lunch break a staff member should go through the

At midday or during the lunch break, one employee should:

- Empty waste receptacles.
- Straighten the magazines and other reading materials.
- Look for smudges on glasstop tables and clean them if necessary.
- Check for spills and clean and disinfect them immediately.
- If there are toys in the waiting area, disinfect them.
- Put furniture back in place.
- Double-check the entryway for tracked-in dirt and clean it if necessary.
- Check for personal items that may have been left behind by patients and remove them.
- Check the restrooms for cleanliness and supplies.

Employees can take turns with midday cleaning. Depending on the office's evening cleaning company, staff may need to also check the reception area first thing in the morning before patients arrive.

**Figure 1.1** Medical Office Cleanliness Tips

reception area to ensure it's neat and orderly. Magazines and other reading materials should be put back in their original places, trash picked up, and waste baskets emptied. You may even need to put the furniture back in its original place. If there are toys in the reception area, they should be disinfected; there are a variety of easy-to-use sprays and towelettes on the market. Depending on the services your cleaning company provides, you may need to do this again at the end of the day and recheck the reception area first thing in the morning. Figure 1.1 is a checklist of cleanliness standards that you can use throughout the day, particularly at midday.

The arrangement of the furniture in the reception area is important. Most experts agree that for every exam room there should be at least 2.5 seats in the reception area. Patients bring family and friends. All the seating should be separate with no couches or love seats; people do not like to share seating, especially with strangers. Figure 1.2 shows a floor plan for a reception area for an internal medicine office where 30 patients are seen each day.

The colors in the reception area should be selected to create a warm, coordinated look. The walls should be painted in calming colors such as light blue or green. Lavender is also considered a calming color. Some soft browns can promote a sense of security as well. Artwork should also be in muted, soft colors. Research suggests that colors affect our behavior. For example, some research suggests that when we see blue, our brains release

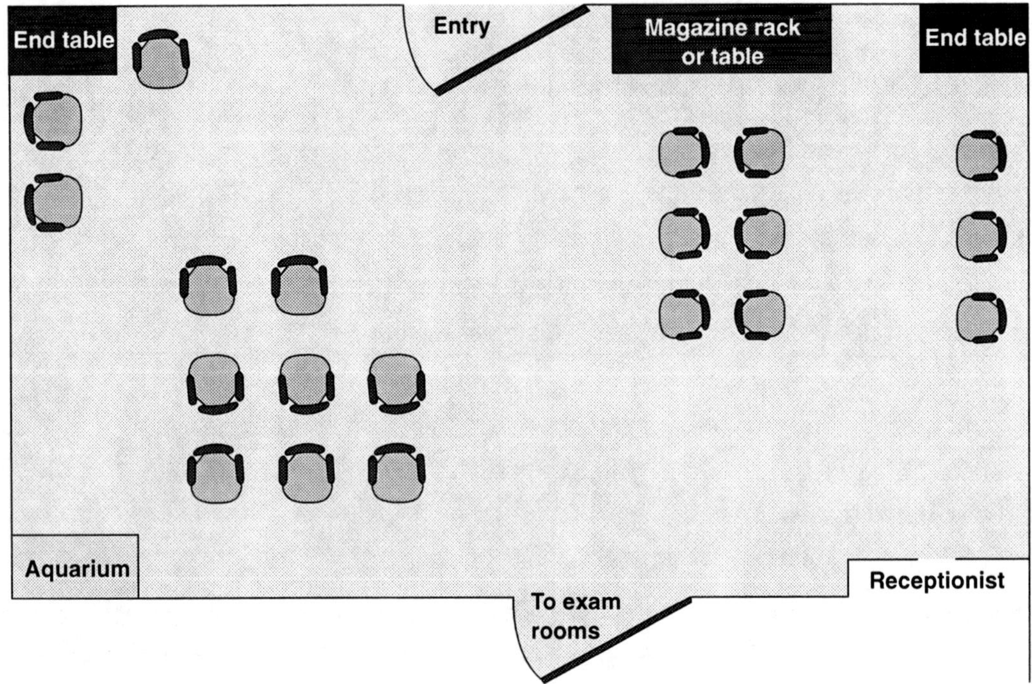


**Figure 1.2** Sample Floor Plan for Internal Medicine Practice

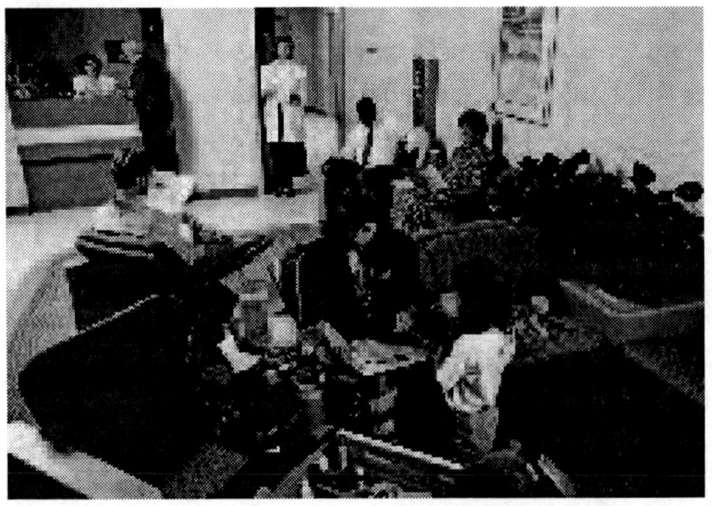

Reception area of a physician's office.

neurotransmitters that relax the body. Green harmonizes and balances, which is why plants in the reception area are appropriate.

The fabric on the furniture and window coverings should also be in the same color family. Remember, bright colors promote a lively atmosphere whereas softer, muted colors create a relaxing atmosphere.

The carpet you choose for the medical office should be a durable style, one that is made to handle a lot of traffic. Throw rugs or scatter rugs should be avoided as they could cause someone to trip and fall. Some offices have a rubber-backed entry carpet to collect dirt as patients enter the office. It is important to have that carpet cleaned or replaced frequently.

Maintaining an appropriate temperature in the reception area is always difficult. Someone is always too cold or too warm. Experts recommend that the area be at 72°F for comfort.

The pediatric office has special needs. If possible, there should be a separate reception area for sick children. Walls should be painted in brighter colors, the artwork should be child focused, and there should be child-sized chairs. Choose toys carefully; items such as blocks and puzzles and books encourage quiet play. Figure 1.3 outlines some ideas for creating a pediatric playroom.

**Reading Materials and Other Distractions.** In a perfect world, patients would be brought back to the exam area within five minutes of arriving in the office. Since that

If the reception area space permits, an area for children to play quietly is an asset.

- If possible, make this a separate area on one side of the reception area. The area should not be close to the entrance/exit of the reception area.
- If there is a television, it should be up high enough that children cannot reach it. Videos should be routinely cycled throughout the day and should be stored behind the front desk of the reception area.
- Toys should be safe and fun, but not encourage active play by the children.
- Toys should be washable. A staff member should take responsibility for ensuring that toys are clean, removing any that need cleaning.
- Books with torn or marked-up pages should be replaced.
- Children's furniture should be durable.
- The area should be situated so that the parents are the prime supervisors, not the front desk staff.
- Educational posters should be placed on the walls.
- Toy boxes, if used, should not have hinged tops as little hands could get caught. A toy box without a top is best.
- All toys should be large enough that they cannot be swallowed.

**Figure 1.3** Pediatric Playrooms

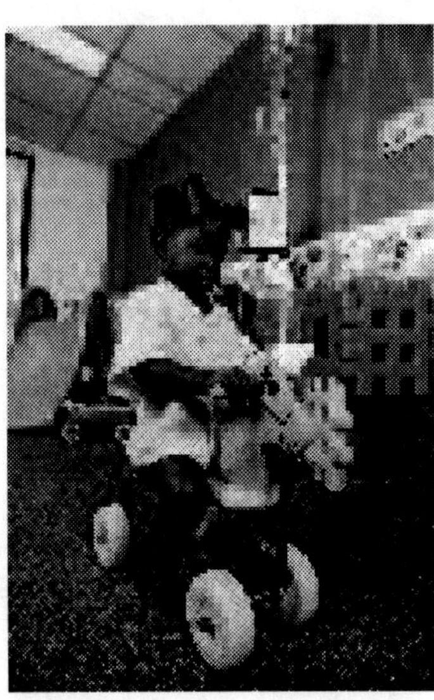

Pediatric playroom area.

doesn't always happen, you need to have the right reading material in the office available for the patients and their families. The magazines should be recent editions (nothing more than six months old) and of interest to the patients. Although it's impossible to have magazines that will interest all your patients, having a variety of news magazines and special interest magazines for your patient population will help. Subscribe to one magazine per topic and choose general interest magazines. For example, if you are going to subscribe to a sports magazine, find a general sports magazine, not a magazine about a specific sport. Magazines about health are particularly good choices, if they are written for the general public and not the medical community. Periodically survey your patients about what magazines they like by displaying the survey in the office. Figure 1.4 shows a sample survey that you could use.

Many offices have a television in the reception area. Be sure it is mounted high on the wall so that patients can't be constantly changing the channel. If the television is turned on, keep it on a station that provides news. Other offices have music playing in the background. Be sure that the music selected is appropriate for your patient population. Remember, both television and music are for the patients, not the staff.

A popular distraction in many offices is an aquarium—it is calming to watch. Unless you have a dedicated staff person who understands the dynamics of maintaining an aquarium, it is best to use a professional service to maintain it.

Educational materials are often found in the reception area. Brochures about various health conditions may be of interest to your patients. You can get these brochures from organizations like the American Heart Association. Be sure to keep only updated materials in the reception area. It is also important that these materials are reviewed periodically

We are interested in finding out which magazines in our reception area appeal to you and also what other magazine topics you would like to see available. Please complete the questions below and return the survey to a member of our front desk staff.

1. I find the magazines in the reception area (check as many as apply):
   _______ are current _______ are in good shape (not torn)
   _______ provide a good selection
2. If you think that the current selection of magazines in our reception area is appropriate, please go to question 4. If you do not think the current selection is appropriate, please continue on to question 3.
3. I would like to see magazines that cover the following:
   _______ sports
   _______ health issues
   _______ family issues
   _______ current news and world events
   _______ children's magazines
   _______ news about celebrities
   _______ other; please list
   _______
   _______
4. Tell us a little bit about yourself:
   I have been a patient in this practice for_______ years.
   I see Dr. ___________ or _________.
   I am ______ years old.
   I am male or female (circle one).

Thank you for your time in completing this survey. Please turn it in to a member of our front desk staff.

**Figure 1.4** Patient Survey

and replaced with newer editions. If you serve a bilingual population, educational materials in your patients' native language are most helpful.

There are a variety of organizations that will provide free or low-cost educational materials. For example, the American Heart Association has a quarterly magazine called

*Heart Insight* that is delivered by mail. The American Academy of Pediatrics has a variety of free or low-cost brochures that may be ordered on its website. Since so many patients are now computer literate, it is worthwhile to do an Internet search to find the most valuable websites for your patients. You can then prepare a list of those websites to hand out to your patients. Chapter 4 discusses how to use search engines to get information you need for your patients.

**Safety in the Reception Area.** We don't tend to think of a reception area as full of hazards, but if we aren't careful, we can create hazards unintentionally. Avoid easily breakable items in the reception area. All furniture should have rounded corners to avoid creating a hazard for small children and older individuals. Artwork should be securely fastened. Any shelves or coat racks should also be securely mounted on the wall.

Avoid anything that may create an allergic reaction or present a poisoning hazard to small children. Use artificial plants and be sure to dust them daily. No candles or potpourri should be used anywhere in the medical office.

If you do choose to have an aquarium, be sure it is built into the wall to avoid the possibility of the aquarium falling or a small child climbing on the tank.

Furniture should be arranged to allow maximum floor space for every patient. Usually, placing chairs along the walls produces the most area. If you need to use the middle of the reception area for additional seating, placing chairs back-to-back may conserve space. Seating should also be arranged so that families or friends may sit together. Room must be available for wheelchairs.

In Chapter 11, we will review overall safety requirements in a medical office. For the reception area, common sense should always prevail when designing and maintaining the area.

**Privacy.** Chapter 7 deals with **privacy** in detail. However, first impressions make a difference. Greeting patients pleasantly when they arrive is important. The sign-in sheet should be monitored closely and names crossed off so that others may not read them. The check-in area should be designed so that patients cannot see computer screens. Every precaution should be taken to ensure that patients are not able to hear discussions about other patients while sitting in the reception area.

**Patients with Special Needs.** There are an estimated 60 million people who are identified as disabled. These disabilities range from having to use a cane or other support while walking, to being 100% blind or needing to use a wheelchair. In 1990 the **Americans with Disabilities Act (ADA)** was passed by Congress. This law requires all businesses to ensure that individuals with disabilities have access to buildings and offices. The reception area of a medical practice should be set up to accommodate patients with

- An entrance must be accessible with ramp and curb cut.
- Both interior and exterior doors must be at least 32 inches wide and easy to open.
- Door handles must be no higher than 48 inches.
- Magazine racks and other amenities must be accessible to wheelchair users.
- Counters and reception stations should be accessible to wheelchair users.
- Space for wheelchair seating in the reception area must be available.
- A restroom must be wheelchair accessible.
- The alarm system must be both audible (sound signals) and visual (flashing lights).
- Accessible handicap parking spaces must be close to an entrance.

**Figure 1.5** ADA Requirements for Medical Offices

disabilities. Additionally, access to the building itself must accommodate individuals who are in a wheelchair, visually impaired, and otherwise unable to access the area. We are all familiar with handicap parking spaces, but there are a variety of other things that your medical office should have in place. Figure 1.5 provides a list of those items that are important throughout the medical office.

## The Intangibles

Attitude is everything! Most people are apprehensive when they come to the physician's office. It is the responsibility of the front desk person to be positive and friendly as patients arrive. You aren't necessarily going to eliminate their fear or apprehension, but you should do nothing to increase it either. It is sometimes easy to forget that the reason patients are in your office is because they don't feel well. They may be cranky, overly sensitive, and sometimes rude. However, you must always maintain a positive attitude.

Many studies have indicated that one of the things that frustrates patients the most is the waiting time. It is important for the front desk staff to maintain communication with the medical assisting and/or nursing staff members who manage patient flow. When the physician is running late, the patients should be advised of the approximate wait time and be given an opportunity to reschedule their appointment. Patients who are scheduled during the period of the physician's delay, but have not yet arrived, should be contacted immediately to inform them of the delay.

Many practices have a standard set for how long a patient should wait before offering a new appointment. If delays become a common occurrence, it is appropriate to review the scheduling process to see if overbooking is the problem.

If a patient or a family member becomes irate and creates a problem, it is best to bring the individual to a more private area. Having another staff member deal with the patient or family member is often helpful. In Chapter 2 you will learn more about how to deal with difficult patients.

## Personal Dress and Style

The medical office is a place of business. Appropriate appearance on the part of the staff goes a long way in reassuring patients that they are in a place where the staff is professional and competent. Many offices have specific **dress codes,** but there are basics in any office. Those basics are shown in Figure 1.6.

If there is no dress code in your office, it is important that you wear conservative business-like clothing to work. Patients will have more confidence in the medical office in general if all staff members are dressed appropriately.

- Your uniform should fit well and be clean and pressed. If it is too tight, obtain a larger size.
- Shoes should be comfortable, white, and in good condition. Open-toed shoes are not appropriate.
- Personal hygiene is very important. Bath or shower every day and use a deodorant. Brush your teeth after every meal.
- Your hairstyle should be conservative in nature. If you have long hair, it should be pulled back from your face. Your hair should be a natural color.
- Tattoos should not be visible to the patients.
- Don't wear perfume or cologne. Many people are allergic to them.
- Body piercing (beyond one set of pierced ears) is not appropriate.
- Fingernails should be manageable working length and the color should be pale or clear. Many offices ban acrylic nails or require that they be kept very short.
- Jewelry should be kept to a minimum.

**Figure 1.6** Basic Office Dress Code

## Summary

As medical office staff, it is important to remember that the patients and their family members are our customers. We must always keep in mind that most patients do not want to be at the physician's office, so it is important to provide a warm, safe, friendly atmosphere. The importance of professionalism in the medical office cannot be overstated. In Chapter 2, we will look at the all-important skill of communication.

# Chapter 2

# Effective Communication

## Introduction

*The medical practice is a business and the patients are the customers. The staff's ability to communicate effectively with patients is critical in providing good patient care. Additionally, the communication between the staff and health care providers is important in the provision of care. What we say, how we say it, and our nonverbal behavior are all forms of communication.*

*We have all had experiences where we were treated rudely or someone's tone of voice or nonverbal behavior has been upsetting to us. Other people's words, tone of voice, or actions can ruin our day or, worse yet, create a conflict. In the medical office, it is important to maintain a professional attitude at all times. This isn't easy, since patients are often not in a good mood because of their illness and our fellow staff members are often overworked. Knowing how to communicate effectively and professionally makes the work environment a more positive place.*

*Many studies suggest that it is not* what *we say, but* how *we say it. These studies suggest that 7 to 10% of how well we communicate is in the actual words, 35 to 40% is in our tone of voice, and 50 to 60% is in our nonverbal behavior. Essentially, how we say what we say is more important than what we say. You probably come into work with a smile on your face and say "good morning" to everyone in a pleasant way and get a positive response from most people. Everyone's reaction is positive because you are positive. However, if you come in with a frown on your face, mumbling "good morning" or, worse yet, saying it sarcastically, you get a different reaction to the same two words.*

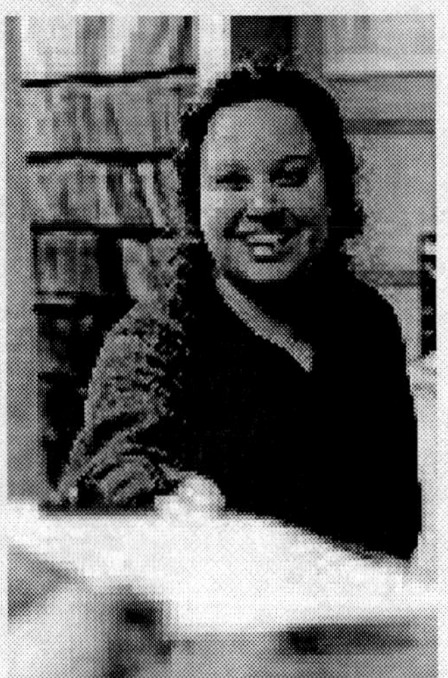

*Our written communication also is an important part of good communication in the office. We will look at the written word in both Chapters 3 and 4. In today's electronic world we have a variety of ways to exchange messages, from emailing and text messaging to chatting online. It would seem that maintaining effective communication would be easy, but we all know it isn't.*

## Chapter Outline

## Elements of Communication

There are four basic elements in any form of communication, whether it is written or oral. The **sender** is the person who sends the information; the **receiver** is the person who receives the information sent. The **message** is the content of the information sent by the sender, and the **feedback** is the response from the receiver of the information. Figure 2.1 illustrates the process.

As you can see by Figure 2.1, communication is a circular process. In the communication process there is a lot of room for misunderstanding. The sender may think he or she has articulated a message well, but the receiver may interpret the meaning differently. The receiver's interpretation is based not only on the words said, but the tone of voice and the body language.

Noise can also interfere in the communication process. In the medical office there are often several conversations going on at once, which may interfere with good communication. Pay specific attention to what external sounds might be interfering in the communication process.

A simple "May I have Jane Little's chart?" can take on a variety of meanings. For example, if a coworker comes up to your desk with a frown on her face while slamming down several other charts on your desk, sarcastically asking for Mrs. Little's chart, she is probably communicating that she is not happy about the circumstances she finds herself in. Is her message that you forgot to get Mrs. Little's chart when you should have, or is she just having a bad day? Your response to her sarcastic request can also increase the tension. If the office is noisy, you may hear the name Lydle instead of Little, further complicating the communication process. If your coworker approaches you with a smile on her face requesting Mrs. Little's chart, you have a different reaction to her request and the coworker is sending a different message.



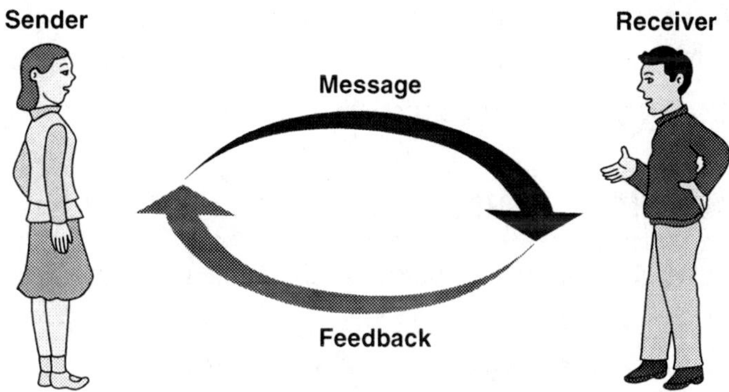


**Figure 2.1** Communication Process

## Communication Styles

Everyone communicates differently. Communication styles are the way people send and receive messages. There are many different ways to categorize communication styles. The way we communicate is influenced by our background, age, and gender as well as culture, education, and the circumstances of the communication. When we communicate, we can be direct or indirect. We might be emotionally open or closed. We might be very passive or aggressive. Most people try to maintain an assertive style, whereas others may be passive-aggressive. For example, aggressive communicators are direct and demanding. Often aggressive communicators insist that things be done their way. Aggressive communicators view life as a competition that they must always win. Passive communicators allow others to make decisions for them and appear uncertain when they speak. Passive communicators never want to make anyone uncomfortable, and they rarely speak up for themselves. Passive-aggressive communicators are often described as manipulators. They are able to appear as if they are uncertain or indirect, but their behavior or their comments are often less than straightforward. Passive-aggressive communicators make snide comments about others. Assertive communicators attempt to be direct but sensitive, looking to make all situations win–win, using compromise and negotiation when appropriate.



A quick search of the Internet using the keywords "communication styles" will provide you with a variety of simple tests to see what your main communication style, however labeled, might be. It is important to recognize that communication styles will differ among people. It is also important to recognize that we don't all communicate in the same style all the time. There is no one best way to communicate all the time, but there are certain principles that will make communication more effective.

The purpose of communication is to get your message across clearly so that it is understood by the receiver. The process can be full of error and misinterpretation. This can cause confusion, wasted time, and sometimes unnecessary conflict. None of us communicates clearly all the time, but there are certain things we can do to improve our communication skills. The next section focuses on some helpful ways to make certain you are communicating effectively in different situations in the medical office.

## Communicating Face-to-Face with Patients

We talk to patients all day, but are we successfully communicating with them? Busy physicians need to get a lot of information in a short amount of time. Because patients often spend more time with the staff than with the physician, it is important that the communication lines are open and working all of the time.

The first step in being a good verbal communicator is to practice thoughtful and clear communication, taking into consideration the receiver of your message. Simplify your language—don't use *myocardial infarction* when completing a medical history with a patient; the patient will know that he had a heart attack, but probably not recognize the words *myocardial infarction.* Don't use medical terminology when common terminology will work.

Next, be sure to speak in a neutral manner, holding back any opinion or emotion that you may have about a particular issue. Sometimes it is important to emphasize certain behaviors with patients, but be careful not to make a judgment about a patient's behavior. For example, a patient with respiratory problems should be encouraged to stop smoking, but should not be told that "people who smoke are just stupid because everyone knows it causes problems." Don't use terms of endearment that may be offensive to some people such as *honey, sweetie,* or *darling.*

Become an active listener. Too often we are so busy figuring out what we are going to say that we are not listening to what the other person is saying. Try to understand what the other person is communicating before you decide what you should say. Listen to hear and understand, rather than to judge. Sometimes it is hard to not tune out when the other person is rambling, but careful listening may help make it a shorter conversation. Figure 2.2 offers some suggestions for good active listening.



- Make the person comfortable. Be sure your body language does not convey a negative message.
- Maintain eye contact. However, there are certain cultures where direct eye contact is not appropriate. Become aware of those cultures represented in your practice.
- Nod when you agree with the speaker, but ask him or her to explain further if you don't understand what is being said.
- Show empathy. Empathetic people listen carefully to others and express concern, but not sympathy or pity.
- Make sure there are no distractions. Don't answer the phone, work on your computer, or do other tasks while speaking with someone. Give the person your full attention. If necessary for privacy reasons, move the conversation into a more private place.
- Don't get emotional—remain calm and pay attention to what the person is saying.
- Be careful if you must disagree or offer constructive suggestions. Don't make the person feel defensive.
- Ask a lot of questions—particularly if you are uncertain of what the individual is trying to communicate.
- *Stop talking.* You cannot possibly be listening if you are talking.

**Figure 2.2** Active Listening Skills

Remember to maintain a professional distance. Becoming friends with a patient or offering to help out an elderly patient with personal tasks is not appropriate professional behavior in the office. Avoid talking to patients about yourself. This makes it easier to keep the relationship on a professional level.

General barriers to effective communication may be found in Figure 2.3. Whenever you have a communication problem, it is important to think about what might have gone wrong. Are the facts not understood? Are the facts being ignored? Are your preheld beliefs getting in the way of understanding the communication? Are you too emotional about whatever the issue is?

There are also special situations where communication may be difficult because of specific physical or mental illnesses or problems. Dealing with the frail elderly or individuals with emotional or mental disabilities requires a great deal of patience on the part of the medical staff. Figure 2.4 illustrates other special situations where good communication may be difficult.

*Defensive behavior.* Sarcastic comments, verbally attacking the speaker, and being judgmental about the subject or the speaker are all defensive behaviors that impair good communication.

*Emotions.* When upset or angry, it is best not to respond or react to the speaker. Wait until you have a clear head to discuss the matter rationally.

*Filtering.* This technique is used when the sender manipulates the information communicated to the receiver. Telling a patient that there is a short waiting time as opposed to saying the physician is behind schedule and the wait will be 45 minutes is an example of filtering. For the sender, 45 minutes is a short period of time. For the patient, 45 minutes may be a very long time.

*Information overload.* Too much information may be distracting for the receiver of the information. The actual message may be distorted and lost in the overload of information.

*Cultural and gender issues.* Although we often approach the communication problems between men and women with a sense of humor, it is important to be sensitive to gender issues in patient care. Also, different cultures may have different meanings for the same thing, thus creating a misunderstanding. It is not expected that you should have an in-depth understanding of every culture represented in the United States. However, if your practice has a significant number of patients that represent another culture, it is a good idea to become familiar with basic customs and cultural differences so that you may communicate well with these patients.

**Figure 2.3** Barriers to Effective Communication

*Patients who do not speak English.* In today's diverse society, this is becoming a more common problem. Although many patients will bring family members with them for the visits, sometimes that is not possible. Also, in some cultures the sharing of bad news is very sensitive and often not communicated. Most hospitals today have access to centralized translation services. Good phrase books are helpful to have also. Speak slowly, do not raise your voice, and avoid using slang. Speak directly to the patients so that you can see one another's facial expressions. Use pictures if necessary.

*Patients with hearing impairments.* There is a wide range of hearing loss in patients today. Patients with complete hearing loss have usually adapted and make use of sign language or interpreters. The bigger challenge comes with patients with a partial hearing loss, usually older people, who may not have accepted their hearing loss. Talk directly to these patients. Speak slowly and raise your voice a little. Remember that privacy is also important.

*Patients with visual impairments.* Many people who are visually impaired have made the adjustments necessary. Be sure to identify yourself by name, speaking in a normal tone. Always let the patients know what you are doing. Alert the patients before you touch them. Explain any machine sounds before they happen. Be sure to tell the patients when you are leaving the exam room and knock before entering the exam room.

*Patients with speech impairments.* As our population ages, we are likely to see more patients who have speech impairments because of a stroke or other illness. Allow these patients time to communicate. Don't rush conversations. Provide them with a notepad to write questions if they would like. Be aware of your own body language and facial expressions.

*Patients who are addicted to drugs or alcohol.* These patients are particularly difficult to deal with as they are often irrational if they are still under the influence. If they are in withdrawal, they are often aggressive and rude. Keep your communication professional, speaking in a calm voice. Follow your regular duties with these patients and do not make judgments.

*Patients who are grieving.* Patients who have suffered the loss of a loved one or who are terminally ill themselves offer a challenge for the medical office staff. It is important to practice active listening with these patients, allowing them to express themselves. Try to understand what the patients are feeling so that you may offer consoling comments. Sympathy and pity are not appropriate.

**Figure 2.4** Challenging Communication Situations

## Communicating with Coworkers, Providers, and Other Professionals

We tend to focus on being good communicators with our patients and sometimes forget that communication within the office is just as important. Because we often spend more time with our coworkers than our family, it is easy to see how poor communication can sometimes lead to complications.

It is easy to laugh and talk with our coworkers throughout the day—it helps the day go by more quickly. However, there is a fine line between having an enjoyable day at the office and letting personal conversations interfere with getting the job done. Lots of loud talking or laughing can lead to the appearance of an unprofessional office. Treating your coworkers with respect and practicing active listening with them are important. All of the skills used in communicating with patients are just as important in communicating with your coworkers.



Conflict in an office is inevitable. The old saying "If you can't say anything good about someone, don't say anything at all" has a lot of value. If you find yourself in conflict with another staff member, do some self-reflection first. Could you be contributing to the problem? Are you rude and abrupt with this staff member? Do you filter information so that he or she gets only part of the necessary facts? Do you talk about the employee with other staff members? If you honestly think that you are not contributing to the problem, then take some time to speak to the person about the problem, engaging your active listening skills. See if you can come to some agreement.

However, there are times when the friction between staff members must be dealt with by the office managers and supervisors. This is never an easy task for anyone. If the situation has become so uncomfortable that patient care is affected, it is important to bring the situation to management's attention. You may not like the solution that the management team comes up with, so be prepared to state your position calmly and effectively. Too often in these kinds of situations, we become defensive when we should not. Be ready to accept that you may need to change your style in order to arrive at a compromise.

What if the communication problem is between you and a member of the management team? Again, it is important to examine your behavior first to see if you are contributing to the problem. At some point, you may need to schedule a meeting with the manager and ask what may be the problem. Remember to use active listening skills. Too often, when we are in conversations with supervisors and managers, we become defensive. The reality is that there are managers and supervisors who need to develop their communication skills as well. Hopefully, you will be able to present your issues clearly and work out the problems. However, you must recognize that at some point you may need to make a decision to look for another job.

If the communication problem is between you and your supervising physician or provider, you have a difficult situation to resolve. The reality is that you may have to modify your communication behaviors to meet the needs of the physician or provider. If the physician or provider has difficulty communicating and creates problems in the office, the management team should work with him or her to resolve the issues. However, sometimes the physician or provider is the manager and is unwilling to recognize his or her own poor communication skills. Again, it may be necessary to look for another job if the situation holds no hope for improvement from your perspective.

The physicians and other care providers in the office are dependent on the staff for information to provide quality patient care. Clearly written messages are critical. Additionally, if you have responsibility for placing any information about the patient in the chart, readable notes are very important.

Keep in mind that proper **etiquette** requires that the physician be addressed as *doctor.* If the physician has given you permission to call him or her by first name, do not do so in front of patients and other visitors to the office.



## On the Telephone

In most businesses, including medical practices, the telephone is a central part of the activity during the day. Each medical practice will have it own policies about how to screen and direct calls, but there are some basic guidelines for good telephone etiquette. Most medical offices have a large volume of calls coming in on a daily basis, so managing those calls is vital to the success of the practice.

First, always answer the telephone in a pleasant manner. If you are wondering how you sound, put a mirror by your telephone so you can see your face. Although it is a visual image, if you have a distressed or angry look on your face, the chances are you are sounding the way you look when you answer the telephone.

The standard rule is that the telephone should be answered within three rings. Sometimes you must answer the telephone and ask the patient to hold, as you are managing several different calls. Be sure to wait for the caller's permission to put him or her on hold. In the event that you are managing several calls at the same time, be sure to get back to all callers if they are on hold for more than one minute. This is often difficult as you may have callers who want to talk on and on. You may need to respectfully put them back on hold in order to keep all callers satisfied that they haven't been forgotten.

Hold the mouthpiece about an inch from your mouth. Speak in a normal tone. Eating or chewing gum while answering the telephone is not appropriate. Be sensitive to the noise around you, as it may affect the caller's ability to hear you. Many offices have headphones for staff members who spend most of their time on the telephone. Do not use a speaker telephone, as you may be violating privacy.

Determine the reason for the call and handle it as directed by your medical office's policy. Be sure to use the patient's name. Depending on the type of call, it may be necessary to repeat the information the patient gives you to determine if you understood what the patient said.

Be patient with the caller. This is not always easy because patients often ramble on about their problems. You may have to ask to put them on hold so that you can respond to other calls. Remember that they are probably calling because they don't feel well. When we don't feel well, we often don't communicate well!

Document messages carefully. The date and time are important, but getting the correct information is more important. Be certain to verify phone numbers and names. If the patient is calling regarding medications, make sure you write down the correct medication in the message. You may have to ask the patient to spell the name of the medication, just to be sure.



In most medical practices, the only calls that are put through to the providers immediately are calls from other providers. Each office will have its own policy about how other calls are to be routed. Table 2.1 shows a sample medical office call routing system.

**Table 2.1** Sample Telephone Call Routing System

| Type of Call | Physician or Other Provider | Take a Message | Clinical Support Staff (Medical Assistant, Nurse) | Business Office Staff or Other Administrative Staff |
|---|---|---|---|---|
| Progress report from patient | | ✓ | | |
| Prescription refills | | ✓ | | |
| Appointments | | | | ✓ |
| Another physician | ✓ | | | |
| Hospital calling for orders | ✓ | | | |
| Patient complaints | | | | ✓ |
| Third-party request for information | | | | ✓ |
| Patient with questions about medical care, test results | | | ✓ To determine if physician needs to speak to patient (abnormal test results) | |
| Patient with billing and/or insurance questions | | | | ✓ |

Most practices have established policies about when telephone calls will be returned. Some offices use the lunch hour; others the end of the day. Some physicians set aside specific times during the day to return calls. Most practices let patients know when to expect a call back from the provider. We have all played the telephone tag game; however, privacy laws (see Chapter 7) take precedence when leaving messages on voice mail.

Cell phones are in common use everywhere. Your personal cell phone should be either turned off or on vibrate during the time you are in the office. You should never take a cell phone call while you are at work. Also, your personal calls coming into the office should be limited to emergencies only. Many offices have signs posted asking patients to turn off their cells phones as well.

Most telephone calls are routine, but when a patient calls with a need for emergency services, proper handling of the call could save his or her life. Depending on the nature of the practice and the nature of the emergency, your office will handle this type of call differently. If a telephone call involves an emergency, stay calm. Depending on your office policy, you may be required to get information (see Figure 2.5) and then either route the call immediately to the physician or put the caller on hold and dial 911. You may also instruct the patient or caller to dial 911 to request emergency services, depending on office policy and the nature of the call.



1. Remain calm.
2. Obtain the following information and be certain to write it down:
   a. caller's name
   b. caller's relationship to the patient (if it is not the patient calling)
   c. patient's name
   d. patient's age
   e. as complete a description of symptoms as possible
   f. the patient's location (address) and phone number
   g. any treatment that has been administered
   h. repeat the information back to the caller
3. Depending on the answers to the above questions and your practice's protocol, you may need to put the patient on hold to call 911. If you are uncertain, consult with the physician or other provider.
4. Depending on the office protocol and the patient's symptoms, you may need to instruct the patient to go to the nearest emergency room.

**Figure 2.5** Handling Emergency Calls

Ultimately, all telephone calls should be handled courteously. Patients should be made to feel that they are important to the practice. Many practices have telephone scripts for the staff so that answers to patients' questions are consistent. This is a great training tool for new staff members responsible for answering the phone.

## Dealing with Conflict



In our world, life is not without conflict. Dealing with angry patients or angry friends or relatives of patients, angry coworkers, or other individuals is a challenge. Handling angry patients is particularly difficult because you are dealing with individuals who are ill and consequently are not in complete control of their emotions. Dealing with angry coworkers or other people is just as difficult. This is where your communication skills will be put to the test.

A fair amount of research supports the notion that angry customers or patients will tell at least two to four times as many people about their dissatisfaction with a business than patients or customers who are happy with the care or treatment they received. Therefore, it is important to handle these angry patients and family members with great care.

Disagreements among staff members in the office are going to happen. How they are resolved is what will determine whether or not your practice is a good place to work. Since you will be with these people day in and day out, it is important that tension between co-workers be reduced whenever possible.

Some people believe that all conflict is inherently bad. Most psychological experts would agree, however, that *within limits,* some conflict may be necessary in order to identify problems and issues among groups, whether at work or at home. If a situation is creating

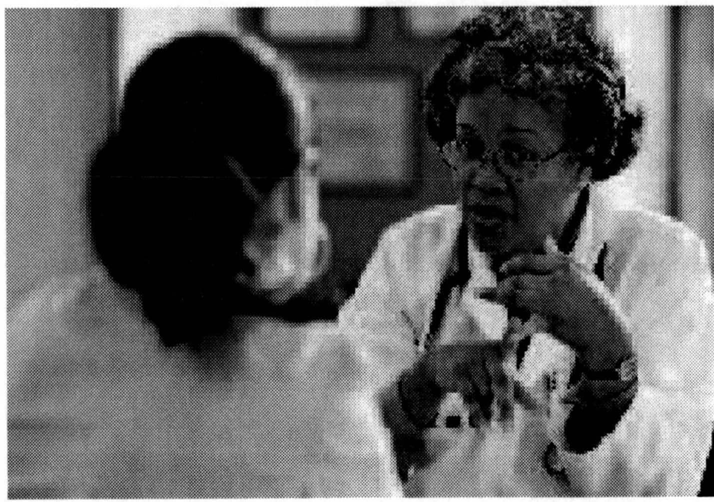

Two medical office employees arguing

1. Empathize with the person. Use a phrase like "I can see that you are concerned."
2. Offer to help the person. "Let's see what we can do to work this out together."
3. Get the facts. Be sure to repeat the facts as you understand them.
4. Don't interrupt the person—let him or her finish.
5. Offer a solution. If you aren't in a position to solve the problem, make sure the person understands that you are not the one who will solve the problem, but you are the person who will follow up to ensure that the right person is aware of the problem. Be very specific with the angry person.
6. If agreement is reached on a solution, repeat the action you are going to take and the time frame in which you are going to take the action.
7. Be certain that the person acknowledges the action you are going to take and the time frame so that there are no further misunderstandings.
8. Follow up as appropriate.

**Figure 2.6** Hints to Handle the Angry Patient



tension and discomfort, it should be recognized and steps should be taken to reduce the tension and stress. Chapter 12 talks about stress more specifically and provides some techniques for managing stress and conflict in the workplace.

Dealing with upset patients is a skill that usually improves over time. Figure 2.6 contains some helpful hints about how to handle the angry patient. The techniques outlined are useful whenever you are dealing with anyone who is upset.

## Nonverbal Communication

All of the previous information should help you improve your verbal communication skills with both patients and the staff in your office. The research on nonverbal communication and behavior began in 1872 when Charles Darwin published *The Expression of the Emotions in Man and Animals.* As mentioned at the beginning of this chapter, most studies suggest that up to 90% of our communication is in how we say something along with our nonverbal cues. Those behaviors and tones may send a contradictory message about what we are actually trying to communicate. An abundance of research has been published on nonverbal communication. Most of the research focuses on seven areas: paralinguistics, facial expression, gestures, eye contact, appearance, body language, and proxemics.

The technical term for vocal communication that is separate from actual language is **paralinguistics.** It is our tone of voice, pitch, inflection, and loudness. We all recognize that the tone of our voice when speaking can change the meaning of our intended communication. A simple example of how tone of voice affects the interpretation of a message was mentioned earlier. The phrase *good morning* can contain a variety of meanings, depending on how it is said. When we speak in a hesitant tone of voice, we may be implying that we are uninterested or we disagree or we aren't understanding.

Tone of voice should be neutral for the most part; this does not mean monotone, however. You can be enthusiastic and expressive to emphasize your point, but be careful not to use a tone that could potentially convey different meanings. Tone of voice is particularly important while on the telephone, as the caller has no body language to view to help interpret your message. Recognize that you will not always have perfect tone of voice, but be conscious of it. Also be aware of how loudly you may be speaking. Do not assume that people can't hear you.



Facial expression is an important part of communication. For example, a smile or a frown can affect how your message is interpreted. Your face may show anger, fear, happiness, or sadness. Try this experiment. In an informal conversation with friends, close your eyes and listen to the conversation. Does the meaning change when you can't see them speaking? That is why listening carefully on the telephone when speaking with patients is so important. You do not have the advantage of also seeing their face to help your understand their message. We read people by the look on their face. Facial expressions in most cultures are fairly similar, but gestures may vary from culture to culture.

Gestures are those movements and signals that communicate without words. We wave and we point. Gestures have different meanings in different cultures, so it is important to become sensitive to those cultures represented in your practice so that you don't unintentionally insult someone. For example, in some Southeast Asian cultures, it is not appropriate to use the "come here" gesture of stretching out your arm and using your fingers to indicate that you want them to come to you. This gesture is considered an insult. In America we cross our fingers for good luck, but in some cultures that is seen as a profanity.

Eye contact is an important part of communication and is often misinterpreted. In American culture, not looking others in the eye may be viewed as trying to hide something. On the other hand, too much eye contact may be seen as intimidating. Many cultures view direct eye contact as inappropriate, particularly between a man and a woman. Looking at another person can indicate a whole range of emotions from hostility to interest and affection. We know when people look away from us when we are speaking that they are probably not listening to us. So how much eye contact is the right amount? Although it is always situational, some communication experts suggest that intervals of four to five seconds are appropriate. Many of us unconsciously already do that when we are listening intently.

Our appearance may speak volumes about us. In Chapter 1 there are suggestions for appropriate dress in the office. However, as illustrated in that chapter, appearance is more than just being dressed appropriately. Our personal hygiene and our choices in makeup and other body-enhancing items send a message. Some of our choices are generational in nature. Younger people are more inclined to have body piercing or tattoos, or both. For some of the older generation, numerous tattoos and piercing are seen as representing the criminal element of society. What one person perceives as sloppy, another sees as fashionable. For the office, conservative dress and appearance are a safer choice.



A 1976 book by Julius Fast titled *Body Language* created a set of interpretations about body language. Although these interpretations became ingrained in our culture, subsequent research suggests that body language may not be as indicative of our feelings and attitudes as was once thought. For example, there is a widely held belief that if your arms are crossed in front of your body, you are angry or frustrated. You may just be in a room that is cold, and you have your arms crossed to preserve body heat. It is widely assumed that a weak or limp handshake is the sign of a weak or timid person. It may just be that the person has arthritis and is unable to grasp anything with a strong grip. When we see someone slumped in a chair during an office meeting, we assume they are bored. They may just be tired or find that position more comfortable. Although our body language and posture may be sending a message, it might be important to confirm our interpretation by the person's spoken words.

**Proxemics** is the study of the amount of space we need around us, our "comfort zone." We perceive that space as belonging to us. When that space is invaded by another person, a communication problem may occur. The amount of distance we need and the amount of space we perceive as ours are determined by a number of things. The situational factors, our social and cultural norms, personality characteristics, and the level of familiarity are all part of how we determine when someone has invaded our comfort zone. The amount of space needed is dependent on the situation. When having a casual conversation with another person, the acceptable space is between 18 inches to 4 feet. However, much of the care we provide patients invades that 18-inch guideline. That is why it is always important to explain to the patient what you plan to do before you do it. This should make the patient less anxious about what is going to happen.

Every day we respond to hundreds of nonverbal behaviors and cues. While verbal and written communication skills are important, much of our response is keyed to the nonverbal behaviors. However, it is important that we don't focus on only one nonverbal behavior or cue. Instead, look for whether the words being said match the nonverbal behaviors. You must consider the situation and the context of the communication. There are situations where more formal behaviors are required. Those same behaviors in an informal setting would be interpreted differently. For example, in a meeting with your supervisor, you probably sit up straight and attempt to stay focused on what your supervisor is saying by maintaining direct eye contact. You listen carefully and try to not show any nervousness. If you were to do that in a casual conversation at a friend's home, it would probably be interpreted very differently. Your supervisor would be happy that you appeared to be paying attention, while your friend would be worried that something was wrong. A single gesture or facial expression may mean any number of things, or the gesture or expression may mean nothing at all. The key is to look for a group of nonverbal behaviors to help you determine what the person is trying to communicate. Table 2.2 summarizes the various types of nonverbal communications.



**Table 2.2** Types of Nonverbal Communication

*Paralinguistics*—the vocal communications that are separate from actual language. This includes our tone, loudness, inflection, and pitch.

*Facial expression*—the appearance of our face as we listen to another speak. Facial expressions may show a range of emotions.

*Gestures*—deliberate movements we make when we speak.

*Eye contact*—looking at another person. The eye contact may indicate a variety of reactions to what is being communicated by the sender.

*Appearance*—our choices about our appearance provide another form of nonverbal communication.

*Body language*—our posture and our movements. Subject to much misinterpretation, our body language may sometimes provide subtle cues about how the message is being said or received.

*Proxemics*—the study of the personal space a person requires for his or her "comfort zone" while communicating. This personal space is situation dependent.

## Summary

We communicate all day long. Sometimes we are effective communicators, and other times we are poor communicators. Here are some skills and practices that will help you be a positive communicator:

- Listen to understand. Make sure that others know you are listening carefully.
- Acknowledge problems rather than ignore them. Work to resolve the problems whenever possible.
- Ask questions and don't make assumptions.
- Give feedback when things are going well. It is always easy to criticize. Work on being positive.
- Use "I" statements to communicate what your concerns are. Don't blame others.
- Pay attention to nonverbal signals, particularly when they contradict the words being said. Don't overinterpret a single nonverbal behavior. Look for a group of nonverbal behaviors to help interpret the message. Watch your own body language.

Some people are just more effective communicators. However, you can build your skills by paying attention to those who do it well and learning from them. By noticing how others effectively communicate, you can improve your communication skills.

Chapter 3

# Writing Basics

## Introduction

*In today's fast-paced world, we speak in abbreviations and acronyms, we write more emails than letters, and we seem to have varieties of the English language being spoken, often at the same time. Good grammar and style in our written communications seem to be forgotten. However, our written word is important because it demonstrates our professionalism to patients, health care providers, and others whom we interact with on a day-to-day basis. In this chapter, we will review the basics of style and grammar. It is not intended that all the rules and guidelines regarding style and grammar be covered here. Every office should have at least one good reference book.* The Gregg Reference Manual, *10th edition, by William A. Sabin is an excellent source of information not only for grammar and style but also for usage and formatting.*

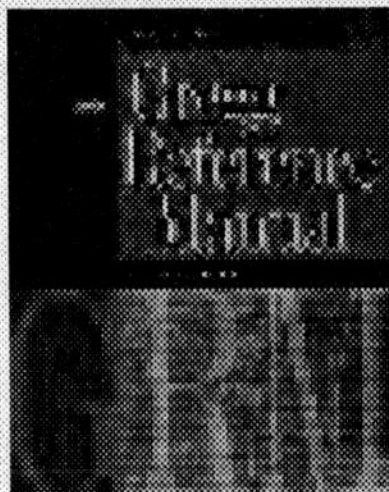


*The Gregg Reference Manual.*

*At the end of this chapter, you will find a variety of examples of letters and memos that could be used in the medical office. In Chapter 4, we will cover email style and etiquette.*

## Chapter Outline

# Grammar

## Nouns (Subjects) and Verbs

One of the most common errors found in writing is the lack of subject (noun) and verb agreement. Sometimes the error is in the proofreading of the sentence, but other times it is because the writer ignored the *noun* (the person, place, thing, quality, or idea) or *subject* of the sentence. You may remember back in English composition that you learned about singular and plural nouns and verbs. The basic rule of agreement is that the verb should agree with the subject of the sentence.

For example, *the number of patients coming today are surprising* is incorrect. The subject (noun) in this sentence is *number,* not *patients,* so the correct grammar is *the number of patients coming today is surprising.*

This rule of subject–verb agreement is the basic rule, but there are exceptions. Table 3.1 illustrates some of those exceptions.

**Verbs.** A *verb* is the part of speech that expresses action or a state of being. In this short section, we are going to look only at some common errors in using verbs. If you are concerned about a specific tense or use of a verb in a sentence, it is best to consult a good reference manual.

**Table 3.1** Subject–Verb Agreement Exceptions

| Exception | Incorrect | Correct |
|---|---|---|
| Subjects joined by *and* (both) | John and Sally is going to the lab. | John and Sally are going to the lab. |
| Subjects refer to one thing or person | The owner and manager of the practice are Dr. Smith. | The owner and manager of the practice is Dr. Smith. |
| Subjects preceded by each or every | Every medical assistant and nurse are coming to the meeting. | Every medical assistant and nurse is coming to the meeting. |
| Subjects joined by *or, either . . . or, neither . . . or* | Either Dr. Jones or Dr. Allen are in charge of the schedule. | Either Dr. Jones or Dr. Allen is in charge of the schedule. |
| When the subject is *you* | You has an infection. | You have an infection. |
| When using phrases such as *along with* or *in addition to, including* | Dr. Weiss, along with the nursing staff, were delayed by traffic. | Dr. Weiss, along with the nursing staff, was delayed by traffic. |

When writing, use the active voice when the subject of your sentence has performed an action. Use the passive voice when the subject is the one who received the action. Here is an example:

*Active voice* Several physicians *reviewed* the lab results.
*Passive voice* The lab results *were reviewed* by the physicians.

In the first sentence, the subject is a group of individuals who have performed an action. In the second sentence, the subject is the lab results that received the action. Using the active voice usually conveys more energy. Whenever possible, use the active voice as it is usually more concise.

Often when we write, we are not clear in our time sequence. In answer to the question "How long has Anna worked at the hospital?" the use of verb tense can mean many different things. Look at the three answers that follow:

Anna worked at the hospital for two years.
Anna has worked at the hospital for two years.
Anna had worked at the hospital for two years.

These three sentences all convey a different meaning. In the first sentence, the past tense used indicates a completed action. Anna no longer works at the hospital. The second answer conveys that Anna has worked at the hospital for two years and continues to work at the hospital. The last sentence tells us that something else may have happened to Anna after her first two years at the hospital. For example, Anna had worked at the hospital for two years when she was asked to work at the new outpatient center.



When writing policies and procedures for the office, it is important to pay attention to the verb tenses to ensure that they are consistent. Here is a portion of a financial policy for patients that has verb tense problems.

> Your insurance policy is a contract between you and your insurance company. We are a participating provider in a number of national health insurance plans. We will bill those plans that we *participated* in. You *were* expected to cover your deductible and copayments and noncovered services. We *made* every effort to inform you of services that may not be covered, but each insurance company is different and the covered procedures do change. In the event your insurance company denies a claim for noncovered services, you will be billed after we receive that denial. Payment *was* expected in 30 days unless other arrangements are made.

A patient reading this policy would be confused about the practice's policies because of the change in verb tenses illustrated in italics. The sentence beginning *We are a participating provider* is followed by a sentence that is in the past tense—*participated*—leading to confusion about whether or not the provider is still participating in the plans.

## Pronouns

**Pronoun–Antecedent Agreement.** *Pronouns* are used in place of nouns and are used to refer to nouns. Pronouns have *antecedents*—the words or phrases that the pronouns refer to in a sentence. In the examples that follow, the antecedent is shown by an *A* and the pronoun by a *P.*

*Incorrect* The physician gave their approval.
A P

*Correct* The physicians gave their approval.
A P

Pronouns must have antecedents and they must agree in number, person, and gender.

*Incorrect* The practice gave their employees a year-end bonus.
A P

*Correct* The practice gave its employees a year-end bonus.
A P

## Pronoun Shift in Point of View

The point of view of a pronoun should not be shifted. The pronouns are italicized in the examples that follow:

*Incorrect* When *I* arrived at work, *you* could see that the waiting room was full.

*Correct* When *I* arrived at work, *I* could see that the waiting room was full.

*Incorrect* *One* should eat fresh fruits and vegetables if *they* want to be healthy.

*Correct* *One* should eat fresh fruits and vegetables if *one* wants to be healthy.

## Indefinite Pronouns

*Indefinite pronouns* refer to nothing or no one in particular. They may be singular or plural. There are some indefinite pronouns that are always singular and that always take singular verbs. Table 3.2 lists those pronouns. Here are some examples:

*Incorrect* Each physician perform the same test.

*Correct* Each physician performs the same test.

*Incorrect* Either Joan or Shannon are on-call this weekend.

*Correct* Either Joan or Shannon is on-call this weekend.

**Table 3.2** Indefinite Pronouns

| All of these indefinite pronouns are considered singular, therefore a singular verb should be used in the sentence. |
| --- |
| Anyone |
| Anybody |
| Anything |
| Each |
| Either |
| Everyone |
| Everybody |
| Everything |
| One |
| Neither |
| No one |
| Nobody |
| Nothing |
| Someone |
| Somebody |
| Something |



## Run-On Sentences

Have you ever listened to someone who talked on and on and never seemed to stop and who couldn't stay on one topic but would shift to another without taking a breath and all the while you are wondering if he or she will ever stop talking? The preceding sentence may be an overblown example of a *run-on sentence,* but since we sometimes write like we speak, it is important to proofread our written work. You will be checking for a variety of errors, including run-on sentences.

A *fused sentence* occurs when two or more sentences are connected to each other without any punctuation such as a comma, a conjunction, a semicolon, or a period. Here are two examples:

*Incorrect* We hope this helps you understand your charges as always our priority is providing the best health care for our patients.

*Correct* We hope this helps you understand your charges, and as always, our priority is providing the best health care for our patients.

*Incorrect* I believe that I do not require further information at this time and I am prepared to proceed with the recommended treatment.

*Correct* I believe that I do not require further information at this time, and I am prepared to proceed with the recommended treatment.

Another common problem with run-on sentences is called *comma splicing.* This problem occurs when two or more complete sentences are separated by a comma alone when other punctuation or a conjunction should be used. A *conjunction* is a connecting word. There are coordinating conjunctions—*for, and, nor, but, or, yet,* and *so.* There are also subordinating conjunctions like *since, if, when, while, even though, although,* and *because.* Here are some examples of correct and incorrect usage:

*Incorrect* She saw the patient, she went to greet her.

*Correct* She saw the patient, so she went to greet her.

*Correct* She saw the patient. She went to greet her.

*Correct* Payment should be made at time of service because this helps keep overall costs lower.

*Correct* Payment should be made at time of service. This helps keep overall costs lower.

## Double Negatives

*Double negatives* occur when the meaning of a verb is negated in one sentence. Only one negative expression for each idea in a sentence is appropriate. Here is an example:

*Incorrect* I did not buy no syringes from the supplier.

*Correct* I did not buy any syringes from the supplier.

*Correct* I bought no syringes from the supplier.

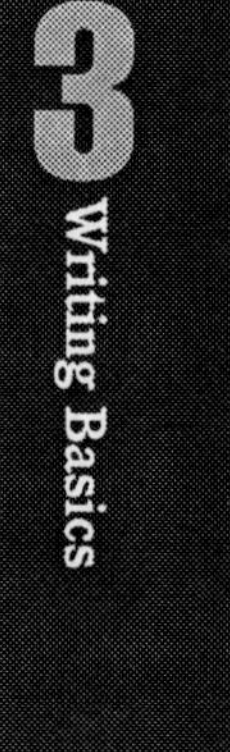


## Dangling and Misplaced Modifiers

*Modifiers* are words describing nouns, verbs, or adverbs. The location of a modifier in the sentence determines what is being described. *Dangling modifiers* are words or phrases that modify the wrong word in sentence. Here is an example of a dangling modifier:

*Incorrect* Having eaten too much chocolate, the patient's stomach began to hurt him.

*Correct* The patient's stomach began to hurt him after he had eaten too much chocolate.

*Correct* Because the patient had eaten too much chocolate, his stomach began to hurt him.

Modifiers are misplaced if they do not communicate the intent of the writer. Because of where the modifier is placed, they can result in humorous or confusing interpretations.

*Incorrect* By using drugs, Dr. Smith was able to treat the patient.

*Correct* Dr. Smith was able to treat the patient with drugs.

*Incorrect* After 16 hours of labor, Dr. John Smith performed a C-section.

*Correct* Dr. John Smith performed a C-section after the patient had been in labor for 16 hours.

*Incorrect* After having been proved incompetent, Dr. Jones admitted the patient.
*Correct* The patient was found incompetent, so Dr. Jones admitted the patient.

## Comma Usage

*Commas* are used to separate clauses in compound sentences, to separate three or more items in a series, after introductory expressions, and in many numerical expressions including dates. Here are some examples of correct usage:

Mrs. Smith said she would be late for her appointment, and she indicated that her husband would be accompanying her.

The patient said she ate fruits, vegetables, meat, and milk at every meal.

Because the patient has problems with allergies to cats, she does not want to be around animals.

On Wednesday, February 13, 2008, all appointments will be canceled.

## Capitalization

The purpose of *capitalization* (or uppercase letters) is to give specific significance to a common noun. Because of that, we sometimes overuse capitalization. The following represents the important situations where you should use uppercase letters:



- Cities, states, countries, languages, nationalities, races, and religions
- The first word of a sentence
- Political groups, official organizations
- Days of the week, months of the year, religious occasions, and holidays
- Eras and historical events like World War II or the Great Depression
- Titles of books, movies, television shows, magazines, articles, songs, and poems
- The word *I*
- Titles that appear in front of person's name
- Brand names of drugs

## Apostrophe Usage

*Apostrophes* are used to show possession or to show the omission of letters. In showing possession, the guidelines are as follows:

- Add *'s* to the singular form of the word to make it possessive:
  - The patient's appointment
  - The physician's schedule

- Add *'s* to the plural nouns that do not end in *s*:
    - The children's books
- Add *'* to the end of plural nouns that end in *s*:
    - Four friends' bicycles

Apostrophes are also used in contractions. A word, or a set of numbers, in which one or more letters (or numbers) have been omitted is called a *contraction.* The apostrophe is used to show this omission. Here are some examples:

- Shouldn't = should not
- I'm = I am
- Don't = do not
- Didn't = did not
- '70 = 1970

*Its* and *it's* are often confused. *Its* is a possessive pronoun meaning "belonging to it," as in *the practice management team made its decision. It's* is a contraction for "it is," as in *It's a busy day for Dr. Smith.*

## Commonly Confused Words

There are words that have the same sound, but different spellings and different meanings. Some words have very similar spellings but mean different things. The following are some of the most commonly misused words:

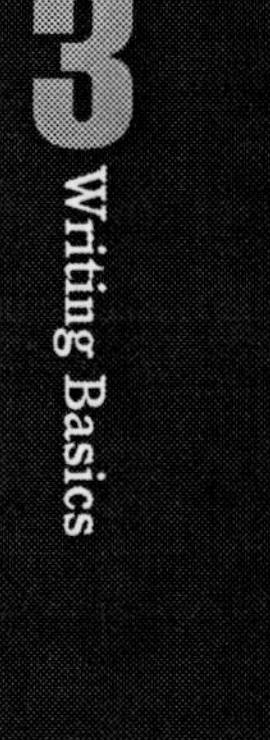


| | |
|---|---|
| **accept/except** | *accept* is to receive<br>*except* is excluding |
| **adapt/adopt** | *adapt* is to change<br>*adopt* is to make your own |
| **adverse/averse** | *adverse* is unfavorable<br>*averse* is reluctant |
| **affect/effect** | *affect* is to change or influence<br>*effect* is the consequence or result |
| **all ready/already** | *all ready* is everything is ready<br>*already* is something has occurred previously |
| **cite/site** | *cite* is a summon before a court of law or a proof<br>*site* is a location |
| **course/coarse** | *course* is a subject in school<br>*coarse* is rough |
| **hole/whole** | *hole* is an opening<br>*whole* is complete |

| | |
|---|---|
| **lose/loose** | *lose* is to misplace<br>*loose* is not firmly fastened, not confined |
| **passed/past** | *passed* is went by<br>*past* is an earlier time |
| **personal/personnel** | *personal* is private, done in person<br>*personnel* is employees or staff |
| **right/write/rite** | *right* is correct, proper, or privilege<br>*write* is to form letters<br>*rite* is a formal ceremony |
| **their/there/they're** | *their* is belonging to them<br>*there* is in that place<br>*they're* is they are |
| **to/too/two** | *to* is toward, a preposition<br>*too* is also, excessive<br>*two* is one more than one |
| **whose/who's** | *whose* is belonging to whom<br>*who's* is who is |
| **your/you're** | *your* is belonging to you<br>*you're* is you are |



### Names and Titles

One of the most common errors in grammar in the workplace is the inappropriate use of titles. Use *Mr., Mrs.,* or *Ms.* before a last name only if the person does not have a degree. Otherwise, use his or her degree. Here are some examples:

*Incorrect* Mrs. Susan Tyndall, CMA
*Correct* Susan Tyndall, CMA
*Incorrect* Dr. Marsha Cook, MD
*Correct* Marsha Cook, MD, or Dr. Marsha Cook

## Effective Writing

The staff members in the medical office are busy with a variety of tasks throughout the day. Often the written documents do not receive the attention that they should. Written documents illustrate the staff's professionalism, and so everyone should ensure that the readers receive the right message. Whether it is a letter to a patient, an insurance company, a hospital or other institution, or the practice staff, care should be taken in the preparation of that communication.

There are three steps to effective professional writing. First, think about the purpose of the written document. Is the letter or memorandum (memo) necessary, or could you make a telephone call instead? What is the purpose of the communication? Do you want to inform the reader or ask for information? Is it to propose an idea or change? Who is the reader? What does the reader want or need? How much does the reader already know? Do you expect a reply to your communication? Identify the key points you want to cover in the communication. What action do you want the reader to take as a result of reading your document? Is it necessary to be specific about that action?

Once you have done your preparation, you have to write the communication. Keep the reader in mind. Although not necessary for all written communication, an outline may be necessary to help organize your thoughts. For example, a short letter to a patient reminding him or her of an appointment does not require an outline. The announcement of the medical practice's new location probably does. In the case of the announcement of a new location, the reader needs to know not only where the new practice is located, but also why the office is moving, how patients might benefit from the move, and directions to the new office. Writing is not a simple task. However, the language of your communication should be elementary. Some experts suggest that most Americans' reading comprehension is at the ninth-grade level, even with a high school diploma. It is not likely that people will complain that your written word is too simple to understand.

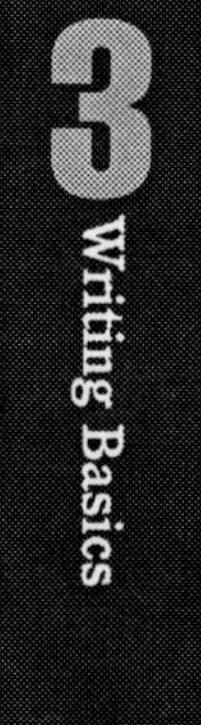


The last step in effective writing is to review, revise, and polish the document. Depending on the document, this may take some time or it may just need a quick review. Table 3.3 is a checklist of things to look for when writing. You may want to add your own items to the list.

In addition to the content of the communication being professional, the look of the communication should also convey professionalism. As an example, many practices have forms that are used to convey lab or other diagnostic results to patients. These forms are mailed to the patient. Often the original blank form gets misplaced, and staff members copy the form from a copy and then a copy of the copy. The end result may be a faded form that looks unprofessional. Keep a file of original blank forms if the practice does not print the form each time it is used.

Throughout this handbook, sample forms and letters are found on specific topics. Here are other sample suggestions that may be of use in the practice.

A formal business letter will be on letterhead. Although preprinted letterhead may be purchased, many practices create a professional letterhead as a template in their word

**Table 3.3** Review/Edit Checklist

1. Is the letter, memo, or other document reader-friendly?
2. Is the purpose of the document stated at the beginning?
3. Are the sentences complete?
4. Do subjects and verbs agree?
5. Have unnecessary words and phrases, as well as professional jargon, been eliminated?
6. Are the facts accurate? Do you have the dates and other numbers entered correctly?
7. Do the sentences flow logically?
8. Have you answered the readers' questions?
9. If action is required by the reader, is the action stated clearly?
10. Is the active voice used more than the passive voice?
11. Are the words spelled correctly and used appropriately? Remember, word processing software will probably catch misspelled words, but it will not catch a properly spelled word used incorrectly.



processing software. The letterhead should contain the name of the practice, as well as the address and telephone numbers of the practice. The business letter itself should have a date, an inside address, a salutation, the body of the letter, a complimentary close, and a signature line. Some business letters also contain a subject line and copy notation. Figure 3.1 contains a sample letter to an insurance company requesting prompt payment of claims.

One of the most difficult letters to write and send is a termination of care letter. The decision to terminate care of a patient is not taken lightly and must meet the appropriate legal requirements in your state. This letter should be sent certified mail, return receipt, so that you have proof of receipt. Many experts suggest that in addition to sending the letter by certified mail, it also should be sent by regular U.S. mail. If the patient is being dismissed for lack of payment, the likelihood is that he or she has other financial problems and may refuse to sign for any certified mail. Although the practice will eventually receive the notice that the patient has refused the letter, the second letter sent by U.S. mail also serves as notice. A sample letter for termination of care is shown in Figure 3.2.

**XYZ MEDICAL GROUP**
734 Medical Lane, Suite 345
Smithville, TX 77456
Phone (555) 534-7896
Fax (555) 534-6298

January 15, 2009

Ms. Joanna Lexington
Director of Claims Management
Next Insurance Company
Dallas, TX 77892

Re: Slow Payment of Claims

Dear Ms. Lexington:

Our practice has experienced difficulties in receiving payments for services provided to your insured patients. Susan James has contacted your office on a weekly basis to follow up on the nonpayment of claims. Her phone calls have not been returned, nor have we received any written information as to why these claims are not being paid.

As of today, we have 37 claims that were filed properly and are at least 90 days past due. We have not received any information as to the status of these claims. The current amount past due is $38,000. We have attached a list of those claims for your review and action.

Our contract with Next Insurance Company calls for payment of all approved claims within 30 days of submittal. The contract also requires Next Insurance Company to provide us with information regarding the status of claims within 15 days of submittal. We have not been provided information on any claims filed since October 15, 2008.

Your immediate attention to this problem is requested. Payment, or a written explanation of why the claims are being rejected, should be provided to us no later than February 1, 2009.

If this matter is not resolved by February 1, 2009, we will have no choice but to inform our patients that we will no long honor their coverage with the Next Insurance Company.

Sincerely,

William W. Wise, MD
Medical Director
Sent Fed Ex
cc: Susan James

**Figure 3.1** Request for Prompt Payment

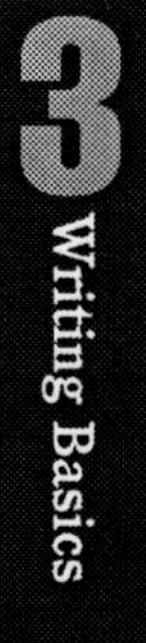

XYZ MEDICAL GROUP
734 Medical Lane, Suite 345
Smithville, TX 77456
Phone (555) 534-7896
Fax (555) 534-6298

CERTIFIED MAIL
RETURN RECEIPT REQUESTED

January 2, 2009

Susan Patient
234 Sunshine Lane
Arcadia, FL 34567

Dear Mrs. Patient:

This is to inform you that I am withdrawing from providing medical care for you effective ______________ *(this should be a reasonable time period based on the patient's condition, but a minimum of thirty (30) days is usually recommended).* I will be available to provide treatment until that date should you require medical attention.

I recommend that you seek care with another physician within the next _____ weeks. If you are unable to locate a physician, please contact the XXXX Medical Society at ______ *(phone number).* The XXXX Medical Society will provide names and contact information of other physicians in the area.

I will make your medical records available to you or to your new physician. Once we have received a written release from you, we will send your record to your new physician. Enclosed you will find a release of information for your convenience.

Sincerely,

William Albright, MD

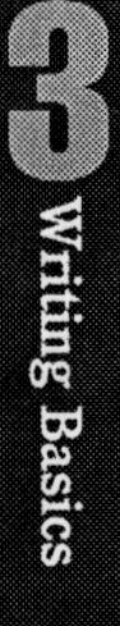

**Figure 3.2** Termination of Care Letter

There is often a need to send out the same letter to a variety of vendors in a less formal way. Figure 3.3 is a sample letter about a change in policy regarding visits by pharmaceutical representatives. The letter would be sent to all representatives. It could also be posted in the reception areas without the specific inside address.

**XYZ MEDICAL GROUP**
734 Medical Lane, Suite 345
Smithville, TX 77456
Phone (555) 534-7896
Fax (555) 534-6298

January 1, 2009

Name of Pharmacy Rep
Name of Pharmaceutical Company
street address
city, state and zip

NEW POLICY FOR VISITS FROM PHARMACEUTICAL REPRESENTATIVES

Beginning January 1, 2009, the XYZ Medical Group will see pharmaceutical representatives by appointment only. We have reserved the hours of 12 P.M. until 1:30 P.M. on Tuesdays and Thursdays for visits.

Please schedule an appointment for your visit. Fifteen minutes will be set aside for you to talk with our physicians. This change will decrease your waiting time to see our physicians.

Thank you for your cooperation.

Carol Worthington
Practice Administrator

**Figure 3.3** General Notification Letter



Memos are written communications within the practice. A memo is not meant to be used for communication with patients, insurance companies, or other outside agencies. Memos should be short and informal communications among the staff and physicians. In small practices, memos sometimes serve as the policy and procedure manual. As a practice grows, more formal policies and procedures may be developed. Email is now often used in place of memos. Figure 3.4 illustrates a memo. Figure 3.5 shows how the same memo might appear as an email. Guidelines about email use in general are included in Chapter 4.

XYZ MEDICAL GROUP
MEMO

DATE: February 1, 2009

TO: All staff and physicians

FROM: James Johnston

SUBJECT: Electronic medical records

Over the next nine months, we will be converting our paper medical records to the electronic medical record (EMR) system. Many of you have been involved in the selection of the software and the implementation of the schedule to convert to EMR.

On Friday, February 8, 2009, there will be a meeting of all staff members and physicians to discuss the implementation of EMR. This meeting will begin at 7:30 A.M. and end promptly at 9 A.M. Patients have been scheduled beginning at 9:30 A.M. that day. Breakfast will be provided. The meeting will be in the conference room.

Thanks for your support of this important project.

**Figure 3.4** Memo Regarding EMR



DATE: February 1, 2009

TO: James Elver, Susan Oliver, Sandy Albright, Christine Smith, John Christian, Paul DeNado, Ranji Sigh

FROM: James Johnston

SUBJECT: Electronic medical records

Over the next nine months, we will be converting our paper medical records to the electronic medical record (EMR) system. Many of you have been involved in the selection of the software and the implementation of the schedule to convert to EMR.

On Friday, February 8, 2009, there will be a meeting for all staff and physicians to discuss the implementation of EMR. This meeting will begin at 7:30 A.M. and end promptly at 9 A.M. Patients have been scheduled beginning at 9:30 A.M. that day. Breakfast will be provided. The meeting will be in the conference room.

**Figure 3.5** Email Regarding a Meeting

## Summary

In Chapter 1, we discussed making a good first impression. Our written communications also make an impression and sometimes are the first thing patients see. A poorly written letter reflects negatively on the practice. Follow the basics when writing—prepare, write, and review. Keep a good grammar and style reference manual in the office, and have others review written documents if you are unsure that you are conveying the right message. Use the review/edit checklist shown in Table 3.3, and add to it to make it a working document for you. Make sure that the written word reflects well on you and your practice.

# Computer Basics and Scheduling

# Part 2

## Computer Basics and Scheduling

# Chapter 4

# Computers in the Medical Office

**Introduction** *We live in an electronic world. Computerized patient information systems, websites, and email play a part in our ability to do our jobs in the medical office. Computers are supposed to make our jobs easier, but sometimes that isn't the case. Whether a patient or an employee, we probably have all experienced when the computers went "down." As employees, we struggled with how to register patients, put in billing information, or communicate through email when the system wasn't working. As patients, we were probably frustrated that the office could not complete a task because the computers weren't working. Having an entire manual system in place isn't a viable option in today's world, but having some information backed up in written form, as well as stored digitally, will be critical when a system fails. Additionally, in the event of a disaster, human-made or weather-related, having the system backed up is critical. Many lessons were learned as a result of Hurricane Katrina.*

*In this chapter, we will review computer basics. We will also explore the management of all the computerized information in the medical office, look at how the Internet can help the practice create some efficiencies, and look at how to use email properly.*

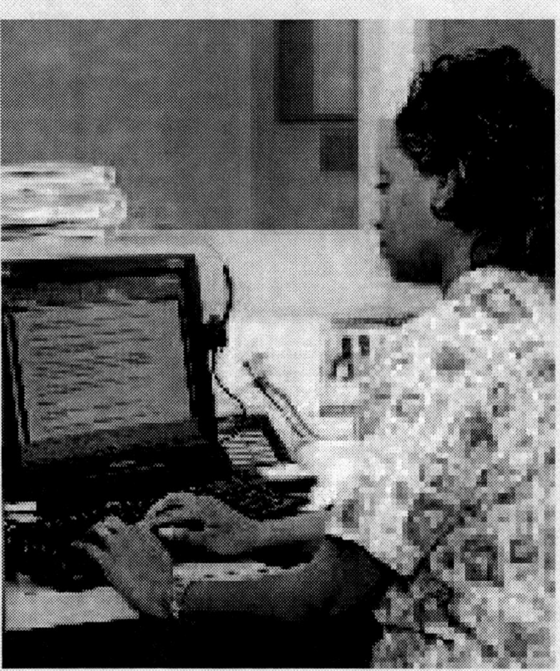

Working at the computer.

## Chapter Outline

## Computer Basics

Computers are used throughout the medical office. Most offices use computers to

- Schedule patients for appointments.
- Post charges and payments.
- Process claims both electronically and in-house.
- Prepare letters and other written communication.
- Check lab results.
- Confirm insurance coverage.
- Maintain medical records of patients.
- Print prescriptions.
- Do Web searches for up-to-date information.

To do all these functions, there is computer hardware and computer software. **Hardware** is a comprehensive term that covers all the physical parts of a computer. Table 4.1 provides

**Table 4.1** Computer Hardware Terms

| Computer Equipment | What Does It Do? |
|---|---|
| Central processor unit (CPU) | This term has two meanings—it is the box that holds the guts of the computer and the chip on the computer that makes everything work. |
| Expansion slot | A connector inside the computer that allows you to plug in a printed circuit board that provides new or enhanced features. |
| Floppy disk | A 3.5-inch square rigid disk that holds data. It is called *floppy* because the earliest disks were flexible. |
| Hard drive | A large-capacity storage device made of multiple disks housed in a rigid case. This device allows the computer to permanently retain and store data. Data may be the operating system, programs, or files. |
| Jump, flash drive, or thumb drive | A device to store files that is removable. Jump drives have taken the place of floppy disks for most personal storage. |
| Keyboard | The name of the primary text input device. |
| Laptop computer or notebook | A battery- or AC-powered personal computer. Notebooks are usually smaller than a briefcase and can easily be transported and conveniently used in a variety of places. |

(*continued*)

**Table 4.1 Computer Hardware Terms** (concluded)

| Computer Equipment | What Does It Do? |
|---|---|
| | They typically weigh less than 5 pounds and are 3 inches or less in thickness. Notebooks are very useful in the wireless environment. |
| Modem | The connection between the computer and the Internet. The modem may connect to a phone line, a TV cable, or a digital subscriber line called a DSL. |
| Mouse | A small, palm-sized pointing device that allows you to tell the computer what to do. On a laptop computer, the mouse is usually an optical device where you move one finger across a designated surface. |
| Optical disc | A high-capacity storage medium that is read by a laser light. In computer terms, a **disc** reproduces data optically with lasers, and a **disk** reproduces data magnetically. |
| Personal digital assistant (PDA) | A small, portable computing device. Depending on the type, you can receive and send data, receive and send email and messages, etc. PDAs usually contain calendars for scheduling. |
| Port | A connection socket for peripherals for a computer. |
| Printer | Transforms digital information to hard copy. |
| Random access memory (RAM) | The most common type of computer memory. It's where the computer stores system software, programs, and data you are currently using. Unless they are saved, the data in RAM memory may be lost when the computer power is turned off. |
| Read only memory (ROM) | The built-in computer memory containing data that normally can be read only, not written to. The data in ROM are not lost when the computer power is turned off. |
| Scanner | A device that captures images from paper and other hard-copy for computer editing and storage. For example, you could scan lab reports and medical records from another office into the computer. |
| Uninterruptible power source (UPS) | A backup battery source for your computer. In the event of a total power failure, a UPS should have enough charge to power your computer for several minutes, giving you time to save your work and safely shut down. |
| Universal serial bus (USB) | The most common type of computer port used in today's computers. |

common terms and definitions for computer hardware. Computer **software** is a general term that describes all the instructions that are in computer programs. Related terms such as applications, instruction sets, and scripts all fall under the category of computer software. Software is more difficult to describe because it is virtual, not physical like hardware. Software consists of lines of code written by computer programmers to create a computer program. Usually when you buy a software program, it comes on a disc, which is physical, but is often referred to as software because that is what the disc contains. The lines between software and hardware sometimes are a bit blurry. Table 4.2 lists some basic software terms.

**Table 4.2** Computer Software Terms

| Term | Definition |
| --- | --- |
| Backup | An extra copy of a file or disk made to ensure data isn't lost. |
| Boot | To start up the computer. |
| Browser | Internet Explorer, Netscape, and Mosaic are examples of Web browsers. The purpose of a browser is to allow for easy interface to access the information on the World Wide Web. |
| Control panel | To modify system settings and controls, you go to the control panel. |
| Crash | A loss of your data or application. Your computer no longer works correctly, and you may lose any data you have not backed up. |
| Cursor or pointer | The name of the arrow that tracks across the screen as you move the mouse around. |
| Database | An electronic collection of information that may be searched or sorted. |
| Dialog box | An on-screen message box that appears asking for more information before proceeding. |
| Directory (folder, subdirectory) | Allows you to organize files and other folders. |
| Disk space | How much space you have to save files. The greater the disk space, the more files you can keep. |
| Documents | Files you create and edit using a variety of software. The document may be a word processing document, a picture, a Web page, or a photo, as examples. |
| Download | Data are transferred from one computer to another. |

*(continued)*

Table 4.2 Computer Software Terms (concluded)

| Term | Definition |
|---|---|
| Hyperlink | The tool that allows you to move from one Web page document to another. It can be underlined text or a graphic. |
| Internet | A worldwide network of millions of connected computers that share and exchange data, news, opinions, and research results. The Internet is not the same as the World Wide Web (WWW). The World Wide Web is a service that is provided on the Internet. |
| Icon | A small, pictorial, on-screen representation of an object, such as a document, program, folder, or disk drive. |
| Landscape | Printing the page sideways. |
| Menu | A list of commands to select from. |
| Operating system | Software that allows your computer to work by communicating with the hardware. The operating system acts as an interface between program software and hardware. |
| Pop-up menu | A menu that may pop up or down and that does not appear at the top of the screen in the menu bar. |
| Recycle bin | Place where you put files and folders that you may later want to delete. Until you empty your recycle bin, the files stay in the bin. |
| Search engine | Very large databases of websites set up by titles, keywords, and text in the pages of the site. |
| Server | A central computer dedicated to sending and receiving data from other computers on a network. |
| Upload | To send a file from your computer to another through a network. |
| Virus | Small program or script that can negatively affect your computer by moving files, deleting files, using your computer's memory, and causing your computer to malfunction or crash. Opening an infected email attachment is the most common way to get a virus. |
| Window | With an uppercase *W*, Windows is the most widely used operating system for personal computers from Microsoft. With a lowercase *w*, a window is the document on your computer screen. |

Tables 4.1 and 4.2 are just a sampling of the common terms used to describe computer hardware and the functions of computer software. There are a variety of sites on the Internet that may help you become familiar with the various computer terms.

## Practice Management Systems

Most medical offices today use a computerized **practice management system (PMS).** This is specific software written to manage the day-to-day functions of the medical practice. Most PMS software allows users to enter and track patients, schedule and track patient appointments, send out insurance claims and patient statements as part of the collection process, process payments from patients and third-party payers, and generate a variety of reports for both clinical and administrative staff. A PMS may link to an electronic medical record (EMR) system, but it is primarily a management system, not a clinical record.

When a new patient comes into the office, or a current patient moves, changes insurance companies, or makes other changes to his or her personal **demographics,** it is relatively easy to make those changes. Additionally, some PMS software may link with the insurance company to determine eligibility before the patient is seen by the provider.

A primary function of a PMS is to schedule patient appointments. A matrix may be easily created and provide all staff with pertinent information. Most important, a computerized scheduling system allows a variety of staff members to book appointments if they have a terminal at their workstation. This may go a long way in reducing patient frustration. Setting up an appointment schedule is discussed in Chapter 5.

At patient checkout, a staff person enters a set of charges. Chapters 9 and 10 detail the appropriate steps for entering correct billing codes, as well as for filing claims. Claims may be sent electronically. Many practices submit directly to individual insurance companies. However, small practices often use the services of an electronic claim clearinghouse to submit their claims. These clearinghouses commonly maintain connections to a large number of payers. By using a clearinghouse, the practice does not need to establish an electronic connection with each and every insurance company.

If the patient is a cash-paying patient, or the insurance company rejects the claim for legitimate reasons, most PMS software allows the practice to send out patient statements directly or by interfacing to a third party for printing and mailing of statements.

Managing the accounts receivable (see Chapter 10) is always a difficult task in a medical practice. Good PMS software is able to sort unpaid claims by insurance company and days unpaid, allowing the billing staff to work the claims in a more productive manner.

Finally, PMS software can create a variety of informational reports for practice management. For example, group practices generate reports from the PMS on provider productivity. Use of medical supplies and medications can be tracked for more effective ordering of supplies and medications. PMS software may help in determining which insurance companies are slow in paying claims. In addition to standard reports, most PMS software allows for individual practices to set up special reports.

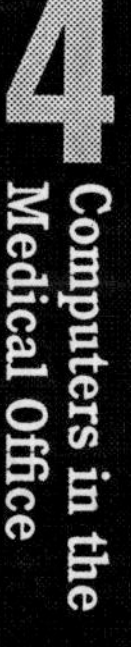

## Electronic Medical Records

The adoption of the **electronic medical record (EMR)** or **electronic health record (EHR)** in the medical practices continues to grow. The two terms EMR and EHR tend to be used interchangeably. An electronic medical record is a medical record in digital format. Although the health care industry as a whole has been quick to use electronic practice management systems and other software for financial data collection, the use of the EMR has more problems associated with its use.

The federal government has a variety of efforts in place to encourage the adoption of EMRs. It is believed that with the widespread adoption of EMRs and other technology we will see fewer mistakes, lower costs, less hassle, and better care. According to the U.S. Department of Health and Human Services (http://www.hhs.gov/healthit/), health information technology (**health IT**) can help prevent many medical errors. The Institute of Medicine estimates that medical errors kill 45,000 to 98,000 Americans each year in hospitals.

When fully implemented, health IT allows comprehensive management of medical information and its secure exchange between health care consumers and providers. Broad use of health IT will

- Improve health care quality.
- Prevent medical errors.
- Reduce health care costs.
- Increase administrative efficiencies.
- Decrease paperwork.
- Expand access to affordable care.

It is also anticipated that not only will health IT improve individual patient care, but it will also bring many public health benefits including early detection of infectious disease outbreaks around the country and improved tracking of chronic disease management.

It is hoped that health IT will help consumers gather all of their health information in one place so they can thoroughly understand it and share it with their health care providers to get the care that best fits their individual needs. Patients will also not have to give their basic demographic and insurance information over and over again in a fully functioning health IT.

There are many issues to be resolved before EMR becomes the standard in this country. The first problem is in actually establishing a standard. The ability of different information technology systems and software applications to communicate; to exchange data accurately, effectively, and consistently; and to use the information that has been exchanged is called **interoperability.** The federal government is attempting to establish standards so that interoperability will exist. Right now, if your practice has EMR, it is possible that the information contained in the EMR is accessible only through your own system. It probably can't be sent to a hospital or other physician's office if those organizations are not using the same software.

The second problem with EMR is cost. Although the costs of some systems for use in medical practices is going down, they are an expense to the practice. Some practices may fear that purchasing a system that does not link to their local hospitals and pharmacies is not a good investment.

Last, designing systems that will work well for the physicians and other providers is not easy, nor is it easy to get physicians and providers to change. There have been several well-publicized failures of installing EMRs in the hospital setting, thus creating hesitation or resistance on the part of many practices.

EMRs and health IT will be an integral part of the medical office in the years to come. Their implementation will take time and will be expensive. They should, however, help save time and provide better care once they are fully implemented.

## Email Etiquette

Since the midnineties, email has been a fixture in all of our lives. Although many people today prefer text messaging, email is a very useful tool in the workplace. We are still developing the proper etiquette for emailing. Although there is no one accepted source for email etiquette, there are some basic principles that are commonly followed.

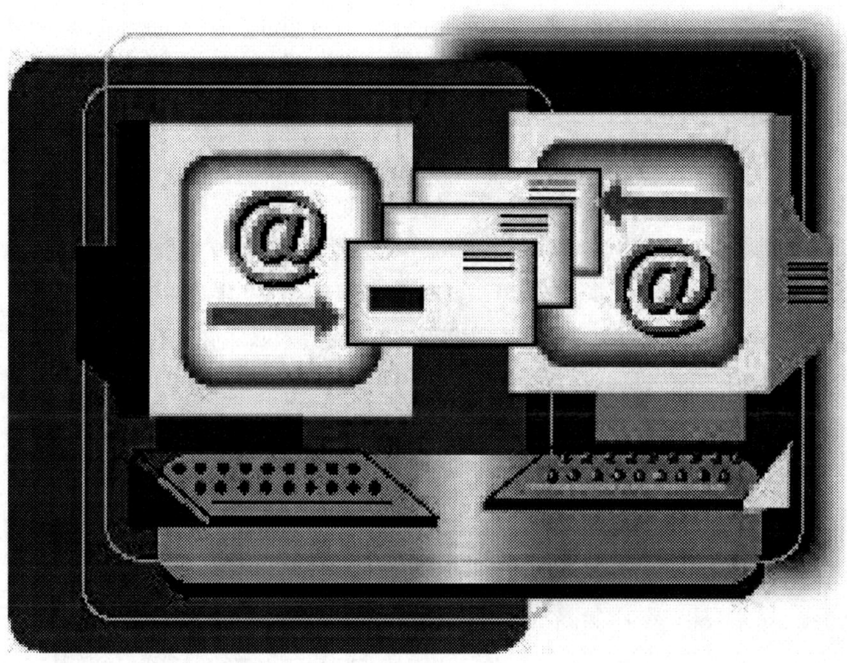

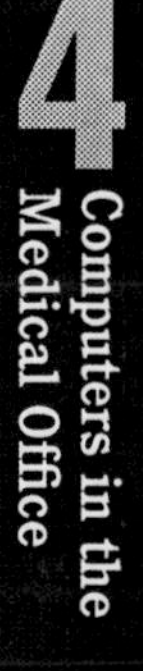

## Addressing Your Email

Email allows you to address your message in a variety of ways. If you are expecting a response from only one person, but want others to know you have sent the email, you use the "To" address line for the person who is to take action. The people on the Cc list are getting the email for information purposes only, not to respond to the email.

The Bcc line should be used sparingly. *Bcc* stands for "blind carbon copy." That means that the recipient—the person in the "To" line of the email—does not know that you are sending a copy to the person in the Bcc line. This should be used rarely.

## Replying to Email

Care should be taken when replying. Using Reply to All can generate a lot of unnecessary emails. As an example, you may be setting up a meeting with 10 staff members. You send out the email, asking that each person let you know if he or she is attending. If the recipients of the email hit the Reply button, that generates only 10 emails. If each recipient selects Reply to All, that generates 90 unnecessary emails.

On the other hand, it may be important to select Reply to All depending on the content of the email. If your response is important to the other people copied on the email, then you should hit the Reply to All button. For example, if the sender is asking for feedback on an idea, using Reply to All may save some meeting time. As a general caution, use Reply to All carefully.

## Formality

Although many consider email informal communication, in the medical practice, particularly with patients and managers, it is important to remember that the email is a written document. You will have to evaluate each situation. A good rule to follow is that if you would normally address a person by *Miss, Mrs., Mr.,* or *Dr.,* then that is the way to initially address him or her in an email. If you normally call the person by his or her first name, you may omit the salutation.

Signatures in email may be important depending on your email system and who you are communicating with in the email. Closing the email with your name, title, and contact information is useful, particularly when communicating with patients.

Some people choose to add a favorite quotation at the end of their emails. Depending on the policies of the practice, you may not be able to do this on business email.

## Content

Because email often becomes a substitute for real conversation, we tend to go overboard with certain things that may not be appropriate in a written conversation. First, emails should be short. If the content requires some length, be sure to use paragraphs to avoid overloading the reader. Be careful with spelling and grammar. Email is a written communication. If you are sloppy in your spelling and grammar, you may embarrass yourself. Be polite—say please and thank you, just like you would in a conversation. Don't use all capital letters for specific words or for the whole message. All caps imply that you are screaming at someone.

There are two other important things to remember about email: Do not assume that your email at work is private. The receiver of the email may send it on to other people, not unlike office gossip. Also, remember that managers and administrators have the legal right to review any and all emails sent and received from the place of business. Don't use your business email for personal communications.

## Printing Emails

One of the purposes of email is to reduce the shuffling of paper. Print out only those emails that require printing—which should be very few. Make use of the file system that exists on your system. Usually, it is called "Folders," so if you must save the email, file it in an electronic folder within the email system instead of printing it.

## Using the Web for Patient Education

Millions of people use the Internet to search out information about health. Studies vary, but it is estimated that approximately 50 to 70% of consumers have used the Net several times to search for basic health information. Many patients show up at the physician's office with copies of all the information they have found about their particular health problem. Knowing what information is valid and what should go in the junk pile takes some knowledge. The U.S. Food and Drug Administration has some helpful hints on its website (http://www.fda.gov/oc/opacom/evalhealthinfo.html). They are summarized in Table 4.3.

**Table 4.3** Evaluating Health Information on the Internet

The following questions and answers are adapted from the U.S. Food and Drug Administration's website to help consumers determine whether websites are reliable and up-to-date.

1. ***Who runs the website?*** A good website makes it easy to learn who is responsible for the site and its information. The information should be found by clicking on the link called "About Us" or "About This Website."
2. ***What is the purpose of the website?*** Is the site to inform you, sell you a product, or raise money? Being able to tell what the purpose of the website is will help you evaluate the authenticity of the information. If the site promises miraculous results, secret ingredients, or uses lots of sensational writing, it probably isn't a valid website for accurate information.

(*continued*)

**Table 4.3** Evaluating Health Information on the Internet (concluded)

3. ***What is the original source of the information on the website?*** Be careful of where the website gets its information. Many sites post information collected for other websites or sources. The original source should be clearly identified. Sites that end in **.gov, .edu,** and **.org** are almost always sources of good information. An **.edu** site run by a university is usually a reliable source. A **.gov** site is a government website such as hhs.gov or floridahealth.gov. Health websites that end in **.org** are not-for-profit groups that are focusing on research and teaching the public about specific diseases or conditions.
4. ***How is the information on the website documented?*** In addition to identifying the original source of the material, the site should identify the evidence on which the material is based.
5. ***How is the information reviewed before it is posted on the website?*** Legitimate health-related websites give information about the credentials of the people who prepare the material for the website.
6. ***How current is the information on the website?*** It is particularly important that medical information be current and updates be clearly posted. If there are a lot of broken links, the likelihood is that the site is not being kept up-to-date.
7. ***How does the website choose links to other sites?*** Reliable websites usually have a policy about how they establish links to other sites. Look for the site's linking policy by clicking on the "About This Website" link.
8. ***What information about its visitors does the website collect, and why?*** Websites routinely track the paths visitors take through their sites to determine what pages are being used. Some health-related websites ask visitors to subscribe or become members. In some cases, this may be done to collect a fee or to select relevant information for the users. In all cases, this subscription allows the website to collect personal information. Any website asking users for personal information should explain exactly what the site will and will not do with the information.
9. ***How does the website manage interactions with visitors?*** There should always be a way for visitors to contact the website owners with problems and feedback. This is usually done through the "Contact Us" link.
10. ***Can the accuracy of information received in an email be verified?*** Carefully evaluate email messages. Consider the origin of the message and its purpose. Many companies use email to advertise their products. The accuracy of health information may be influenced by the desire to promote a product or a service.
11. ***Is the information discussed in chat rooms and blogs accurate?*** Although you may get some good information about specific diseases or disorders, chat rooms may perpetuate misinformation. Most Internet service providers do not verify what is said in chat rooms or blogs, so be very skeptical of information acquired there.

Many practices use the information found on the Internet to create patient handouts. For example, a gastroenterologist might collect information from the quality websites about a colonoscopy to hand out to patients before the procedure. A pediatrician might use the Internet to prepare a handout about vaccinations or overuse of antibiotics in children. Many health organizations like the American Cancer Society or American Heart Association often have quality handouts available for free from their websites. If you do make use of the Internet to create patient education information, be sure to check the websites routinely to ensure that you have the latest updates.

Patient handouts created from Internet sites may be a great time saver for providers. However, it is important to remember that providers still bear a responsibility to explain procedures to their patients under informed consent. Informed consent will be covered in Chapter 7.

## Other Uses for the Web

Many practices today have their own websites. These sites may be used for advertising the practice, providing information about the providers, and allowing communication between the practice and the patients. Many sites provide an opportunity for new patients to either download the new patient registration forms, or to actually do the paperwork online. These can be time-saving devices for the medical office staff.

Additionally, the Internet may be a good source of information for patients about their physicians and hospitals. Most state health or regulatory licensing department websites contain information about both physicians and hospitals. Each state does this differently. It is important that someone in the practice routinely check the state's health or licensing website to ensure that erroneous information is not posted.

## Preventing the Data Disaster

Events like September 11, 2001, Hurricane Katrina, the destructive tornados in the Midwest, the flooding on the West Coast, and various other weather-related and human-caused disasters have made us all think more about planning for disaster. However, something as simple as a cut telephone cable line or a roof leak in your building can lead to problems in the day-to-day operation as well as the long-term viability of the practice. Data security is critical for the success of the practice.

Most, if not all, medical practices back up data every day. Usually done in the off hours, data are either stored to a tape or to another server. The assumption is that the backup will never be needed. That assumption is not a good one, but unfortunately, most practices learn that lesson the hard way.

Every practice should have a backup and disaster recovery plan. That plan needs to consider the following:

- Where are the original software CDs stored? Do you have an up-to-date inventory of the software applications used in the practice?
- How easily can you restore your system if it goes down?
- How often do you test your backup files (i.e., do you test restoring data from the backup on a routine basis)?
- Are you backing up all necessary files? Most practices are great at backing up the PMS and the EMR, but what about your payroll and accounts payable files, your financial statements, and any other clinical databases that your practice uses? If the practice still uses transcription services, are those files backed up?
- Do you have a plan in place in the event of a disaster? Chapter 11 covers the steps to be taken in the event of a pandemic. While developing that plan, the practice should also develop a written plan in the event of a natural disaster. Some of the steps may be different, but the plan is equally important.

A checklist for preparing for the unexpected computer shutdown is found in Table 4.4. Having a good backup plan in place will help maintain the practice in the event of a disaster.

**Table 4.4** Checklist for Preparing for a Computer Shutdown

1. Install and maintain virus scanning software. Scan your network routinely.
2. Maintain telephone line(s) outside your main system that can act as a back door for your practice if the main phone system is disrupted.
3. Purchase a maintenance agreement to help cover the costs of recovery of corrupted files and crashes.
4. Purchase an uninterruptible power supply for phone systems and networks.
5. Use two different carriers for cell phone coverage. This may help ensure coverage when one carrier goes down.
6. House your communication systems in different closets or spaces. This avoids creating a single point of failure for all systems in the event of a roof leak or other building damage.
7. Make sure that employees are able to reach the system through the Internet on their home computers. That way, they can work offsite if your building is shut down for any reason.

## Summary

In a very short amount of time, the medical practice has gone from a "write it once" pegboard system to a paperless medical office. The advantages of computer technology and the Internet are many. They provide us with the ability to store and manage large pieces of information and data. They help us communicate information more efficiently with our patients and fellow staff members. They provide up-to-date information on health-related issues. Most of us cannot imagine life without computers and the Internet. But, for all the advantages of the new electronic age, there are disadvantages. We have added responsibilities in making certain we are prepared with a backup when the human-caused or weather-related disaster occurs. We have to spend time explaining to our patients why information on the Internet is not accurate. Last, we could lose some of the personal touch that is so important in providing quality health care if we are not careful.

# Chapter 5

# Appointments

## Introduction

*We have all heard the stories about the long waits in the physician's office. Maybe as a patient we have been subjected to them also. Managing the appointment schedule is one of the most important functions for the staff of a medical practice. Problems occur when the providers are consistently overbooked with patients or when patients are not scheduled appropriately. Patients become upset and staff members become frustrated when the schedule is not well managed. The efficient and effective scheduling of appointments is critical to the success of any medical practice. The schedule should allow for a productive flow of patients.*

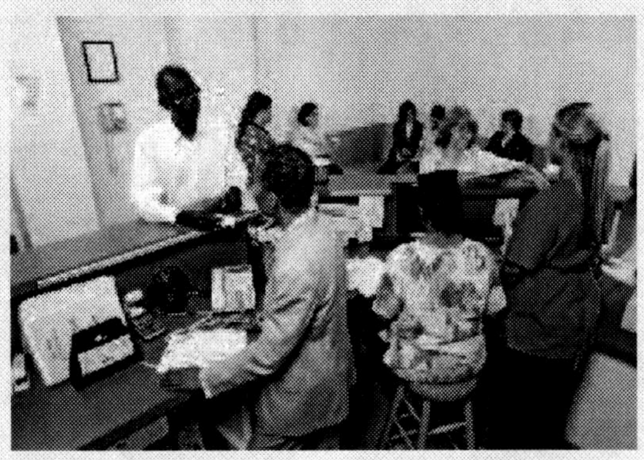

## Chapter Outline

## Appointment Basics

The ideal schedule provides adequate time to see each patient and allows for dictation time, call-backs, and emergencies, not to mention breaks and time for lunch. When designing the schedule, it is important to consider the physician's preferences as well as the patients' needs and convenience. Also, before developing a schedule, it is critical to consider the number of exam rooms available on a daily basis.

All providers' schedules are not the same. Physicians and other providers such as physician assistants (PAs) and advanced registered nurse practitioners (ARNPs) may have different preferences about how patients are scheduled. In large group practices, it is advantageous to get the providers to agree to have similar slots for similar problems. If the practice has several staff making appointments, the more straightforward the schedule, the less likely there will be mistakes. When designing a provider's schedule you need to allow time for the provider to do other things, such as:

- Returning phone calls.
- Making hospital rounds, if appropriate.
- Blocking time for surgery, if appropriate.
- Dictating (assuming there is no electronic medical record in place—see Chapter 4).
- Reviewing lab and other test results.
- Meeting with other physicians.
- Meeting with pharmaceutical representatives and other vendors.
- Performing teaching responsibilities, if the provider is on the staff of a teaching hospital.

Attempting to meet the needs of the patients is difficult. Patients sometimes view their problems as urgent when they are really routine. Other times, the opposite is true. In today's busy world, patients have expectations that may not always be met. The schedule should be designed so that the maximum number of patients may be seen, with the minimum amount of waiting time. Keep in mind that the schedule is always a work in progress. Table 5.1 illustrates some basic questions that should be asked of all patients calling to make an appointment.

Finally, be careful to make the best use of the room resources available. This is often a trial-and-error process. Most practices don't have enough exam rooms. Group practices typically assign a certain number of exam rooms to each provider, depending on the specialty. For example, in primary care, assuming there are an adequate number of rooms, each provider is assigned at least three rooms. One room has a patient who has just had vital signs completed and is waiting to be seen; one room has a patient and the provider

**Table 5.1** Questions to Ask the Patient When Scheduling an Appointment

- What is the reason for the visit?
- How long have you had the symptoms?
- How severe are the symptoms?

Once the reason for the visit is known, it is easier to schedule the patient according to the practice guidelines. If the problem is urgent, then the patient is scheduled for the same day or next day, or possibly directed to the emergency room. Assuming that the problem is not urgent, identify a day for the patient to be seen.

- Ask the patient if he or she would prefer a morning or an afternoon appointment.
- Provide the patient with one or two possible times during that specific day or afternoon.
- Limit the number of choices of time. Providing the patient with a long list of possible times simply increases the time necessary to make the appointment.
- Confirm the appointment day, date, and time with the patient.
- Be sure to enter the appointment in the computer system or on the book.

in it; and the third room has a patient getting dressed to leave. The patient in the third room may be waiting for final instructions from either the provider or the medical assistant or nurse. In a specialty practice, two exam rooms per provider may be adequate as the specialist typically spends more time with the patient. There are no hard-and-fast rules, however. The clinical assistant, whether a medical assistant or a nurse, is responsible for keeping the exam rooms full at all times. That allows the physician or other provider to move from room to room in the most effective way. Offices use various symbols to let the provider know which patient is next. It could be as simple as placing the chart in a certain direction in the chart holder on the door of the exam room, or as complex as using a light signal system for each exam room. Keeping the exam rooms full is sometimes a balancing act because no two patients have the same needs.

## Types of Schedules

There are two types of scheduling tools. For many years, practices relied on a handwritten appointment book and many small practices still do. However, computerized scheduling is a more efficient way to schedule patients—assuming that staff members are able to use the computerized schedule properly.

The benefit to a handwritten schedule is that usually one person is in control of the schedule. That is also a negative feature, however, because if that person is not available, it may be difficult to get the next appointment scheduled.

Using a computerized scheduling package is helpful and saves time. A computerized schedule allows a variety of people to schedule appointments, which is more convenient for the patients. Additionally, the time it takes to set up the schedule book is reduced because you may be able to create a schedule once and have it repeat every day.

To set up a provider's schedule, whether handwritten or computerized, you must establish a **matrix.** A matrix is simply the arrangement of the appointment times available for each provider. If your office is using a handwritten appointment book, the matrix for each day must be entered. In a computerized system, a standard matrix can be entered once and made to replicate wherever appropriate. Figure 5.1 illustrates a sample page from a handwritten matrix. A computerized appointment schedule is shown in Figure 5.2.

The first consideration in setting up the matrix is the type of practice. This is important because it will determine how long each appointment should be. A primary care practice will see more patients in a shorter period of time than some specialty practices. Some physicians are able to see patients faster than others, so establishing a workable schedule for each physician is often trial and error. There is no such thing as a perfect scheduling method, but your first step is determining the time frames. This requires working with the physicians or other providers to establish the times for the types of patients seen.

Once the time frames are established, the type of visit gets an assigned amount of time. The time is established based on the reason for the visit and the physician's preference. Usually, appointments are created in either 10- or 15-minute increments, as illustrated in Table 5.2.

**Table 5.2** Appointment Increments

| Type of Visit | Time | | Time |
|---|---|---|---|
| Short visit | 10 minutes | or | 15 minutes |
| Medium visit | 20 minutes | or | 30 minutes |
| Long visit | 30 minutes | or | 45 minutes |
| Complex visit | 40 minutes | or | 50 minutes |

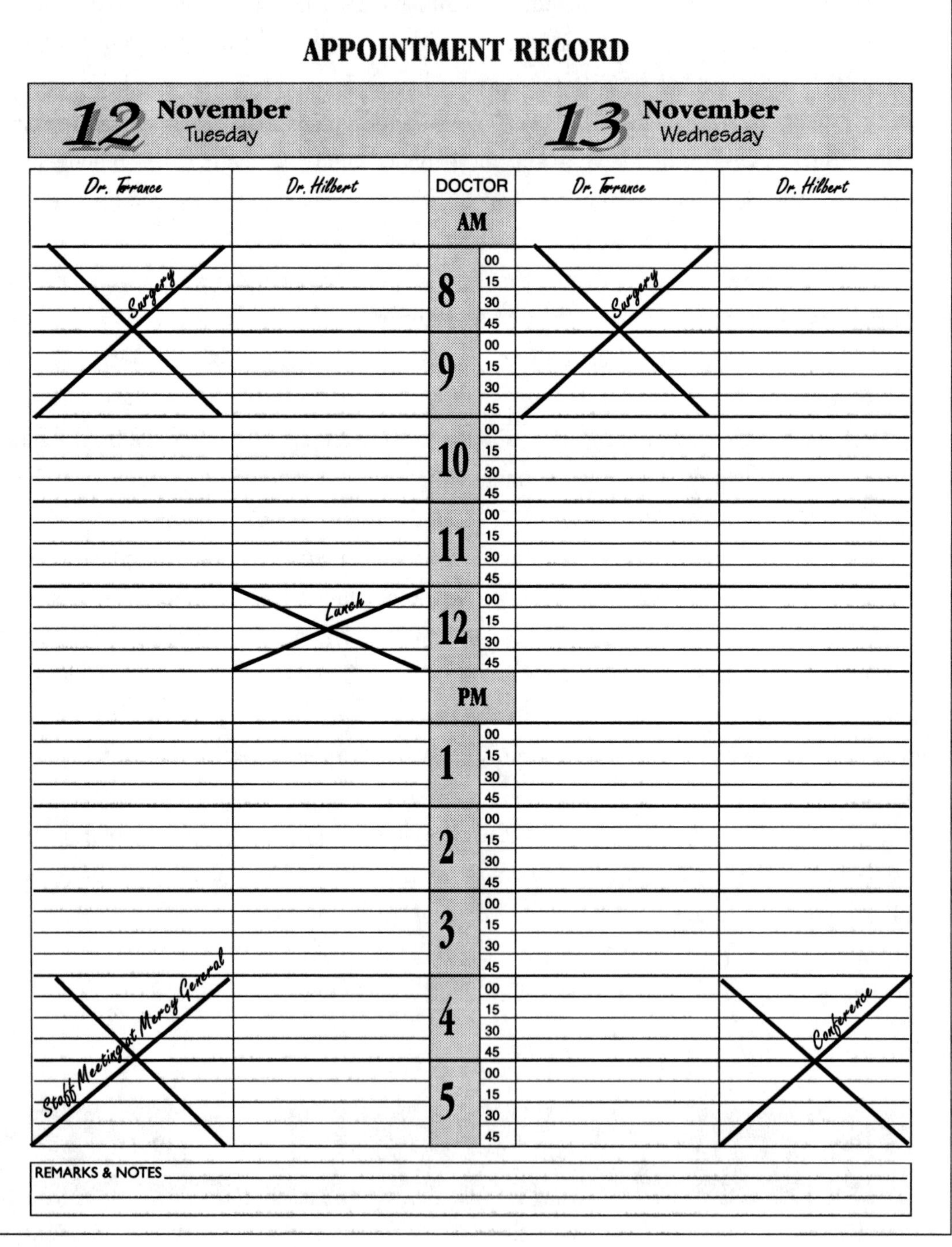


**Figure 5.1** Handwritten Matrix

From Booth et al., *Medical Assisting,* 3e, p. 241. Copyright © 2005 The McGraw-Hill Companies, Inc. Reprinted with permission.

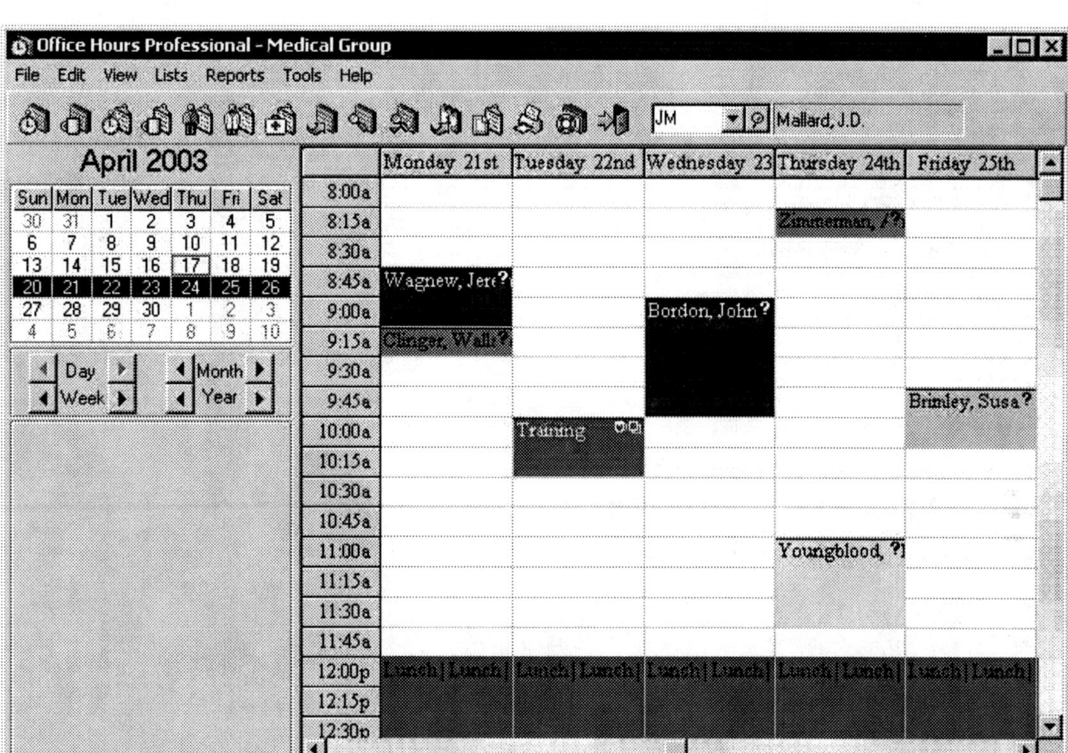


**Figure 5.2** Computerized Schedule

From Booth et al., *Medical Assisting,* 3e, p. 246. Copyright © 2005 The McGraw-Hill Companies, Inc. Reprinted with permission.

The staff scheduling patients should be aware of the amount of time each physician prefers for the presenting problems. Each specialty will determine how much time should be set aside.

Noting the reason for the visit in the schedule is helpful. Depending on the system, you may able to insert a few words. Abbreviations are also useful in this instance, as long as everyone in the office knows the meaning of the abbreviations. Table 5.3 lists some commonly used abbreviations in appointment scheduling.

There are a variety of ways to schedule patients. The method chosen usually depends on the provider's preference. You should regularly review your appointment methods and modify them to ensure a smooth flow of patients with as little waiting time as possible.

## Time-Specified Schedule

This is also known as a *stream schedule.* It assumes a steady stream of patients all day long at regular, specified intervals. Most practices do some version of time-specific scheduling.

**Table 5.3** Common Abbreviations in Scheduling

**BP** or **BP✓** is a blood pressure check
**Can** or **CX** is cancellation
**c/o** is complains of
**CP** is chest pain
**CPE** is complete physician exam
**F/U** is follow-up
**N&V** is nausea and vomiting
**NP** is new patient
**NS** is no-show patient
**pt** is patient
**RE✓** is recheck
**RS** is reschedule
**Rx** is prescription
**SOB** is shortness of breath
Your office may have other abbreviations that are in use as well.

For example, minor medical problems are handled in 10- or 15-minute visits, while physical exams require a 30- to 45-minute visit. Often a minor problem can be doubled-booked with the physical to ensure the best use of the provider's time. Figure 5.3 is a sample of a time-specified or stream schedule.

## Wave Schedule

A traditional wave schedule assumes that some patients will arrive early and some will arrive late. The first step in using a wave schedule is to determine the average time of each patient visit. Then you divide one hour by the average visit time. As an example, if it is determined that patient visits average 12 minutes, then the provider can see five patients in an hour. All patients are told to come in at the beginning of the hour. The physician then sees the patients as they arrive. It is easy to see how this type of scheduling can create problems for both the provider and the patients. A sample wave schedule is found in Figure 5.4.

## APPOINTMENT RECORD

**12 November** Tuesday — **13 November** Wednesday

| Dr. Smith | Dr. Prescott | DOCTOR | | Dr. Smith | Dr. Prescott |
|---|---|---|---|---|---|
| | | AM | | | |
| Hospital rounds (X) | | 8 | 00 | | (X) |
| | | | 15 | | |
| | | | 30 | | |
| | | | 45 | | |
| | | 9 | 00 | | Christine Mitchell OB |
| | | | 15 | | Sara Roberts OB |
| | | | 30 | | Roxanne Johnson OB |
| | | | 45 | | |
| | | 10 | 00 | | Lori Bradley OB |
| | | | 15 | | Susan Case OB |
| Susan Anson FU | | | 30 | | Terri O'Reilly OB |
| Chery Lippett PX | | | 45 | | |
| | | 11 | 00 | | no patients-catch up |
| Terri Jones Consult | | | 15 | | Susan Hayley OB |
| | | | 30 | | Nicki Jones OB |
| Rita Colon FU | | | 45 | | Toni Ramirez OB |
| Phone calls Lunch (X) | | 12 | 00 | | Phone calls Lunch (X) |
| | | | 15 | | |
| | | | 30 | | |
| | | | 45 | | |
| | | PM | | | |
| Phone calls Lunch (X) | | 1 | 00 | | Phone calls Lunch (X) |
| | | | 15 | | |
| Bill Rice New PT | | | 30 | | Kelly Bernard PX |
| | | | 45 | | |
| Joseph Platt FU | | 2 | 00 | | Sarah Houston PX |
| Monique Ramirez FU | | | 15 | | |
| Alan Jonson PX | | | 30 | | Maria Ortega PX |
| | | | 45 | | |
| Carol Morris PX | | 3 | 00 | | Hayley Nicks PX |
| | | | 15 | | |
| Taylor Morris PX | | | 30 | | Phone calls Hospital rounds (X) |
| | | | 45 | | |
| Joy Martinez sore throat×5days | | 4 | 00 | | |
| Thomas Ortega FU | | | 15 | | |
| | | | 30 | | |
| | | | 45 | | |
| | | 5 | 00 | | |
| | | | 15 | | |
| | | | 30 | | |
| | | | 45 | | |

REMARKS & NOTES

**Figure 5.3** Time-Specified Schedule

From Booth et al., *Medical Assisting,* 3e, p. 243. Copyright © 2005 The McGraw-Hill Companies, Inc. Reprinted with permission.

## APPOINTMENT RECORD

| | 12 November Tuesday | | 13 November Wednesday | |
|---|---|---|---|---|
| DOCTOR | Dr. Smith | Dr. Prescott | Dr. Smith | Dr. Prescott |
| AM | | | | |
| 8:00 | Hospital rounds | | | |
| 8:15 | | | | |
| 8:30 | | | | |
| 8:45 | | | | |
| 9:00 | | | | Christine Mitcell OB |
| 9:15 | | | | Sara Case OB |
| 9:30 | | | | Roxanne Johnson OB |
| 9:45 | | | | Lori Bradley OB |
| 10:00 | Susan Anson FU | | | |
| 10:15 | Chery Lippett FU | | | Susan Case OB |
| 10:30 | Terri Jones Consult | | | Terri O'Reilly OB |
| 10:45 | Rita Colon FU | | | Susan Hayley OB |
| 11:00 | Janet Hodge PX | | | Nicki Jones OB, Toni Ramirez OB |
| 11:15 | Joseph Hernandez PX | | | Phone calls |
| 11:30 | Derryn Vance FU | | | |
| 11:45 | Brett Vanguard FU | | | |
| 12:00 | Phone calls Lunch | | | Phone calls Lunch |
| 12:15 | | | | |
| 12:30 | | | | |
| 12:45 | | | | |
| PM | | | | |
| 1:00 | Phone calls Lunch | | | Phone calls Lunch |
| 1:15 | | | | |
| 1:30 | Bill Rice New PX | | | Kelly Bernard PX |
| 1:45 | Joseph Platt FU | | | |
| 2:00 | Monique Ramirez FU | | | Sarah Houston PX |
| 2:15 | | | | |
| 2:30 | Alan Jonson PX | | | Maria Ortega PX |
| 2:45 | Carol Morris PX | | | |
| 3:00 | Barbara Stewart FU | | | Hayley Nicks PX |
| 3:15 | | | | |
| 3:30 | Taylor Morris PX | | | |
| 3:45 | Joy Martinez sore throat x5days | | | |
| 4:00 | Thomas Ortega FU | | | |
| 4:15 | | | | |
| 4:30 | | | | |
| 4:45 | | | | |
| 5:00 | | | | |
| 5:15 | | | | |
| 5:30 | | | | |
| 5:45 | | | | |

REMARKS & NOTES

**Figure 5.4** Wave Schedule

## Modified Wave Schedule

There are many different ways to modify the wave schedule. In the previous example, all patients are told to come in at the beginning of the hour. One way to modify the wave is to tell two patients to come in at the beginning of the hour, with the third patient coming in at 20 minutes past and the last two patients at 20 minutes before the next hour. The theory is that some patients will arrive early and some late and it will all work out that on average five patients will be seen in an hour. Modifying the wave schedule is really a function of the number of exam rooms available. A sample modified wave schedule is shown in Figure 5.5.

## Block Time

This type of scheduling sets aside blocks of times for specific purposes. As an example, an obstetrician-gynecologist might see all the obstetrical patients in the morning and the gynecology patients in the afternoon. An internist might see the diabetic patients for two hours every other day and hypertensive patients from 2 P.M. to 4 P.M. every day. Blocking time is very dependent on the type of practice and the physician's preferences. The sample in Figure 5.3 is both a time-specific and a block schedule.

Many practices double-book a time slot. Late patients, patients who cancel or no-show regularly, and urgent visits are all good reasons to use the double-booking technique. A good scheduler will analyze where double-book slots will work the best.

As you can see, there is no perfect method of booking. Most offices use some combination of the various textbook definitions of scheduling. Scheduling patients is an art. Everything going according to the schedule is usually the exception, not the rule. It is important to pay attention to continual scheduling problems. It may be necessary to rethink the way scheduling is done. It is, however, critical to recognize that some scheduling problems are a result of human behavior, something you may not be able to fix.

Before they leave the office, patients should be given an appointment card if they are scheduled to return for another visit. To reduce error, enter the appointment in the appointment schedule first; then fill out the card for the patient. A sample patient appointment card is found in Figure 5.6.

Finally, the appointment book, whether handwritten or computerized, is a legal document. The records must be kept in accordance with the laws of your state. There is more information about record retention in Chapter 7.

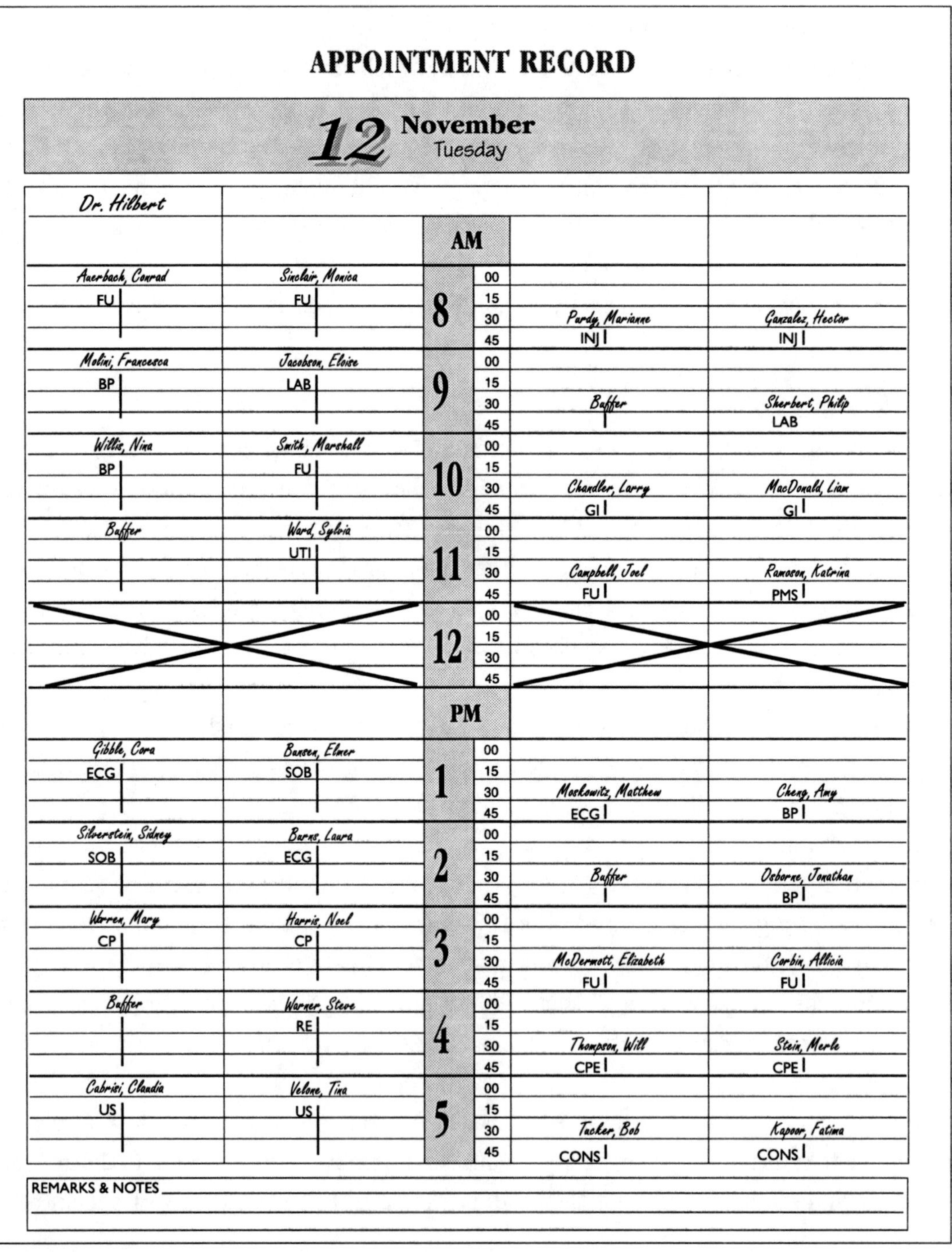

## APPOINTMENT RECORD

**12 November** Tuesday

| Dr. Hilbert | | | | | |
|---|---|---|---|---|---|
| | | AM | | | |
| Auerbach, Conrad | Sinclair, Monica | 8 | 00 | | |
| FU | FU | | 15 | | |
| | | | 30 | Purdy, Marianne | Gonzalez, Hector |
| | | | 45 | INJ | INJ |
| Molini, Francesca | Jacobson, Eloise | 9 | 00 | | |
| BP | LAB | | 15 | | |
| | | | 30 | Buffer | Sherbert, Philip |
| | | | 45 | | LAB |
| Willis, Nina | Smith, Marshall | 10 | 00 | | |
| BP | FU | | 15 | | |
| | | | 30 | Chandler, Larry | MacDonald, Liam |
| | | | 45 | GI | GI |
| Buffer | Ward, Sylvia | 11 | 00 | | |
| | UTI | | 15 | | |
| | | | 30 | Campbell, Joel | Ramoson, Katrina |
| | | | 45 | FU | PMS |
| X | X | 12 | 00 | X | X |
| | | | 15 | | |
| | | | 30 | | |
| | | | 45 | | |
| | | PM | | | |
| Gibble, Cora | Bunsen, Elmer | 1 | 00 | | |
| ECG | SOB | | 15 | | |
| | | | 30 | Moskowitz, Matthew | Cheng, Amy |
| | | | 45 | ECG | BP |
| Silverstein, Sidney | Burns, Laura | 2 | 00 | | |
| SOB | ECG | | 15 | | |
| | | | 30 | Buffer | Osborne, Jonathan |
| | | | 45 | | BP |
| Warren, Mary | Harris, Noel | 3 | 00 | | |
| CP | CP | | 15 | | |
| | | | 30 | McDermott, Elizabeth | Corbin, Allicia |
| | | | 45 | FU | FU |
| Buffer | Warner, Steve | 4 | 00 | | |
| | RE | | 15 | | |
| | | | 30 | Thompson, Will | Stein, Merle |
| | | | 45 | CPE | CPE |
| Cabrini, Claudia | Velone, Tina | 5 | 00 | | |
| US | US | | 15 | | |
| | | | 30 | Tucker, Bob | Kapoor, Fatima |
| | | | 45 | CONS | CONS |

REMARKS & NOTES

**Figure 5.5** Modified Wave Schedule

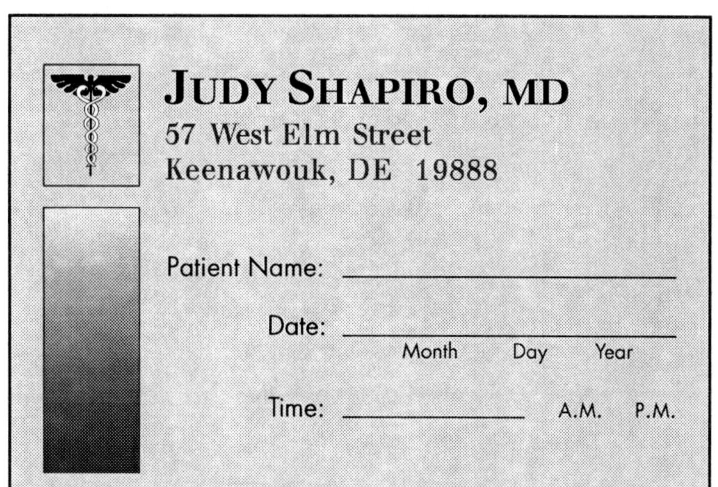
JUDY SHAPIRO, MD
57 West Elm Street
Keenawouk, DE 19888

Patient Name: ______________________

Date: ______________________
Month Day Year

Time: ____________ A.M. P.M.

Figure 5.6 Appointment Card

From Booth et al., *Medical Assisting,* 3e, p. 247. Copyright © 2005 The McGraw-Hill Companies, Inc. Reprinted with permission.

## Patient Reminder

There are two time-honored traditions to remind patients of their appointments—a telephone call and/or a patient reminder card. Both may be effective, but timing is everything. The reminder card should be mailed at least 10 working days before the appointment, and the reminder telephone call should be made at least 2 working days before the appointment. In today's busy world, reminding a patient the day before the appointment may be too late.

Additionally, under the various privacy laws it is important that the telephone reminder and/or card reveal as little information as possible. A script should be used for telephone reminders because often the message is left on voice mail. The script should be very simple. A sample script is found in Figure 5.7.

Many practices have stopped mailing appointment reminder cards due to the cost of postage and the effort needed to complete the cards. If your practice uses appointment

"This message is for (*patient's name*). You have an appointment with Dr. (*last name of physician*) on (*day of week and time*). Please call our office (*give telephone number*) if you have any questions or need to reschedule the appointment."

(*The specialty of the physician should not be provided.*)

Figure 5.7 Appointment Reminder Script

reminder cards, be sure that the minimum amount of information is on the card. Reminder cards are normally used only when appointments are made many months in advance. When a patient is in the office scheduling a follow-up visit for several months in the future, a useful technique is to have the patient address the reminder card. The card then needs to be placed in a **tickler** file and mailed 7 to 10 days before the scheduled visit.

## Scheduling Strategies

We all know that the patient schedule is a work in progress. We hope that all patients arrive on time, call to cancel, and have given the schedulers the appropriate information so that the appointment is scheduled properly. We also hope that the physician doesn't get delayed from hospital rounds and that no urgent patient care issues arise during the day that may cause delays and rescheduling. Since those perfect days are few and far between, here are some suggestions for dealing with common patient behavior that creates scheduling problems.

### Chronically Late Patients

We all know people who arrive late for everything. For those patients who are chronically late, first talk with them and explain that their lateness creates problems for other patients and the physician. However, don't expect a major change in behavior. If the behavior continues, book the patient only for the first appointment of the day, or the first appointment after lunch. Or, you could tell the patient that his or her appointment is for a certain time, but actually schedule it for a slightly later time (i.e., tell the patient 3:00 P.M., but actually book it for 3:15 P.M.). Another technique is to book the patient in a double-book slot. There is no good solution for late patients. Many patients are deliberately late because they know they will have to wait to see the provider.

### No-Show Patients

When a patient does not show up for his or her appointment and has not canceled that appointment, it is important to document that information in the patient's chart. Every office will have a different protocol, but the information should be passed on to the medical assistant, nurse, or physician to determine if the patient needs to be contacted regarding the missed appointment. There may be important medical reasons for the patient to be contacted.

Some patients routinely don't show up and then call and make another appointment. If you have patients who routinely fail to show up for their appointments, you may need to flag their information in your computerized appointment system. You may be able to double-book these patients routinely. By double-booking, not as much productive time is lost when they don't show up.

Some physician practices have started to assess a fee for patients who do not show up and who do not cancel their appointment at least 24 hours in advance. Although this practice is not particularly patient-friendly, it may be necessary to implement this fee in order to better serve your patients that do show up. This type of policy must be clearly stated in writing in the financial policies.

As a final action, physicians can dismiss these patients from their practice. This is always a last resort, but it may be necessary to ensure that the physician's potential liability is covered.

## Patients Who Consistently Cancel Their Appointments

We all have reasons for canceling a doctor's appointment. If a patient does it infrequently, it is usually not a problem. For those patients who routinely cancel their appointments, it is important to first work with the patient to determine if there is a way to modify his or her behavior. Just as with the no-show patient, the canceled appointment information should be passed on to the medical assistant, nurse, or physician to determine if the patient needs to be contacted regarding the missed appointment. There may be important medical reasons for that patient to be contacted.

## Providers Who Are Late

Just like patients, there are some physicians and other providers who are chronically late. I once worked with a surgeon who would call and say he was on his way to the office from the hospital and he would "be right there." The drive between the office and the hospital was 10 minutes. He would consistently arrive at least 45 minutes after he said he would. His staff quickly learned to schedule around this bad habit so that the patients were not inconvenienced.

In surgical offices and in primary care offices where the physicians visit the hospital first thing in the morning, care must be taken to not start office hours at an unrealistic time. Wise schedulers and staff have the exam rooms full for the physician's arrival. Patients should be advised of any delays. Depending on the length of the delay, it may be necessary to reschedule patients.

## Unscheduled Patients

Unless you are working in a walk-in clinic, most medical practices discourage patients from walking in without an appointment. For those patients who do walk in, it is important to get enough information from them to determine if their medical problem warrants being seen by a provider. Usually a medical assistant or nurse can make a quick assessment of the urgency of the patient's problem to determine if he or she should be worked into the day's schedule, scheduled for another day, or sent to a walk-in facility or the emergency room. Every office should have a policy regarding how the walk-in patient should be handled.

### Sales Representatives/Drug Representatives

Throughout the day, your office may be visited by pharmaceutical company representatives, home health salespeople, durable medical equipment salespeople, and clinical lab representatives along with other individuals interested in selling goods to the physicians. Because they are salespeople, they can be very pushy. Patients will not understand why the pharmaceutical representative is allowed to go in to see the physician while they wait in the reception area. It is important that every office establish a policy regarding when outside salespeople will be seen in the office. Once the salespeople know the policy, they will usually follow the rules because they don't want their time wasted either. Many offices post their policy in the reception area so that patients are also aware of the process.

## Appointments with Other Providers

A provider may want to have the patient seen by a physician in another specialty, or have diagnostic tests done. It is also possible that the patients will need to be admitted to a hospital.

In making an appointment for the patient, it is first necessary to know what restraints or requirements the patient's insurance policy may have. You will learn more about **third-party payers** in Chapter 8, but some insurance companies have restrictions on where the patient may go. Your first step is to determine from the insurance company if there are any restrictions. Assuming that you are able to meet those restrictions, you can then begin to set up the additional care needed.

Sometimes physicians want the patient to be seen in **consultation,** sometimes in **referral.** Consultation and referral would seem to be the same thing, but they aren't. In a consultation, the physician is sending the patient to another physician for care with the expectation that once the treatment is complete, the patient will be directed back to the first physician for future care. The first physician expects a letter or phone call from the treating physician to report on the patient's progress. In a referral, the patient's care and treatment is actually being transferred to another physician. For example, a patient diagnosed with prostate cancer by a urologist will have a consulting visit(s) and treatment by an oncologist. Often the urologist will work hand in hand with the oncologist. Once the patient's treatment for prostate cancer is complete, the patient continues to see the urologist for biannual testing for the disease. A family physician may refer a patient with severe diabetes to an endocrinologist for his or her complete care as diabetes affects a variety of organ systems. Although the difference between consultation and referral may seem minor, it sometimes is important to distinguish between the two.

Scheduling a patient for diagnostic tests requires knowledge of the local testing facilities and their policies. The patient needs to be advised of any behavioral restrictions before going for the tests. The most common restriction is no food or water after midnight the day before a test. For some tests, additional preparation by the patient is required. Before a colonoscopy, for example, the patient must engage in a modified fast for at least 24 hours before the test, as well as take preparations that will aid in emptying the gastrointestinal tract. Another example for women is that many radiology centers ask patients not to apply deodorant the day of their scheduled mammogram.

If you work in a surgeon's office, you may be the person responsible for scheduling surgeries. This requires coordination between the hospital or outpatient surgery center, the surgeon's schedule, and of course the patient's schedule. The patient will probably be apprehensive about surgery which sometimes may create a challenge in getting him or her scheduled. Before scheduling any procedure, however, it is important to get **precertification** from the insurance company. There is more discussion about precertification in Chapter 8, but if the patient has any kind of private health insurance, it is likely that precertification is necessary.

Once the precertification is obtained, the clinical assistant contacts the hospital operating room scheduler or outpatient surgery center. Most surgeons have dedicated time set aside for them in the operating room or outpatient surgery center. The scheduler coordinates the surgery time between the facility and the surgeon's schedule. Once the time is set, the surgeon's office is responsible for also scheduling any other preoperative procedures, such as an electrocardiogram (EKG), for the patient.

Most surgical offices have prepared patient packets that provide all the necessary information. Calling the patient the day before is a good procedure to institute. Patients rarely forget that the surgery is scheduled, but they may have questions or concerns about their surgery. Be sure the patients understand that they must have someone drive them to and from the surgery center the day of the surgery.

Although Chapter 8 will cover medical insurance more thoroughly, keep in mind that many patients are in a preferred provider network (PPN) of some kind. When selecting specialists for the patient's referral or consultation, as well as diagnostic tests and surgery, it is critical to ensure that he or she is kept "in network." If for some reason that is not possible, it is the responsibility of the referring physician's office to make sure the patient or patient's family member understands the "out-of-network" referral. The patient may then check into the insurance policies regarding out-of-network referrals.

## Summary

A medical practice needs a well-managed appointment system in order to run smoothly and efficiently. The number of providers, the facility size, and the types of services provided all will influence how the schedule is determined. The schedule may be a simple book or a computerized system. There are several different types of scheduling methods. The front desk staff, working in conjunction with the clinical staff, need to keep the exam rooms full, yet allow time for providers to do other tasks affecting patient care throughout the day. No scheduling system is perfect, so it is important to watch for chronic scheduling problems and work on solutions to those problems. Remember, the perfect scheduled day for the practice will not happen every day!

# The Paperwork

# Part 3

## The Paperwork

# Chapter 6

# Medical Terminology

**Introduction** *Although the support staff members in a medical office do not need to be experts in medical terminology, it is important that everyone have a good understanding of the various medical terms that are used consistently in the office. You must think of medical terminology as a foreign language—one that is easy to learn if you understand how the words are formed. In this chapter, we will cover only the basics. There are several excellent medical dictionaries available. There should be at least two medical dictionaries in the office—one at the front desk and one in the back office.*

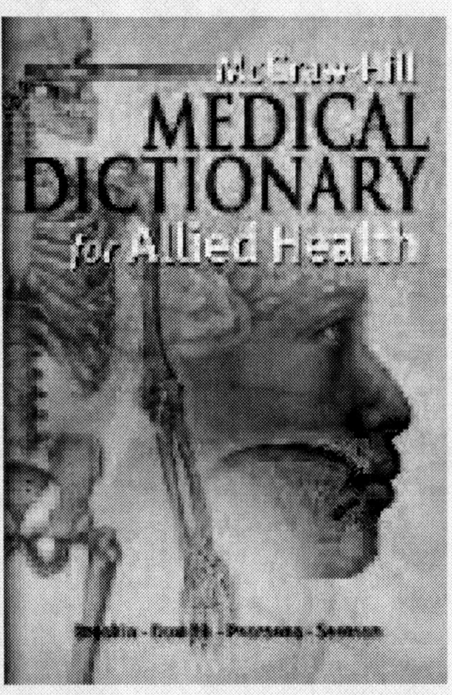


## Chapter Outline

## Prefixes, Suffixes, and Word Roots

Medical terms are made up of prefixes, word roots, suffixes, and combining forms. The basic rules are:

1. A **prefix** is the first part of the word (left of the word root).
2. The **word root** is the part of the word that refers to the anatomy. There can be more than one word root in a medical term.
3. The **suffix** is the last part of the word (right of the word root).
4. **Combining forms** are word roots where a vowel is added at the end of the word root to help make the term easier to pronounce.



Figure 6.1 illustrates how a medical term is put together.

Prefixes are found at the beginning of the word. Not all medical terms have prefixes. Usually, prefixes are not altered when added to the word root–combining form, but there are exceptions. If a word root–combining form begins with a vowel, then a prefix that ends with a consonant is used or the vowel at the end of the prefix is dropped. As an example, *anti-* means against but the word for against acid is *antacid,* not *antiacid.* Table 6.1 contains a list of common prefixes and their meanings.

The suffix of a word occurs at the end of the word. The suffix modifies the meaning of the medical term. For example *-ectomy* is a suffix that means to remove or excise. *Hysterectomy* is a medical term that means removal of the uterus. Some suffixes are stand-alone nouns that can be added to make the medical term more specific. For example, *-mania* can

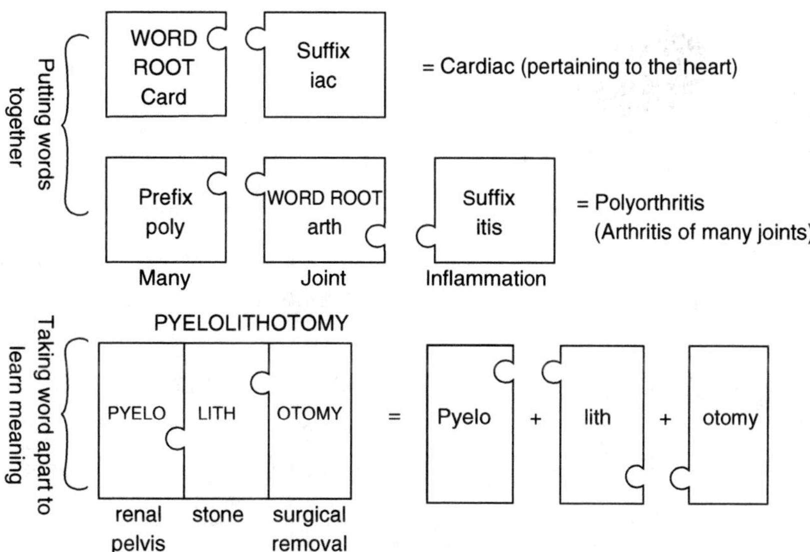


**Figure 6.1** How a Medical Term Is Put Together

stand alone as a word that means an abnormal obsession. However, it may be used as a suffix to describe an abnormal obsession of a specific thing. *Pyromania* is an abnormal obsession with fire. Table 6.2 lists the most common suffixes.



### Table 6.1 Common Prefixes

| Prefixes | Meanings | Example |
|---|---|---|
| **a- an-** | without | *anemia* is a condition in which there is a reduced delivery of oxygen to the tissues |
| **ab-** | from, away from | *abduct* means to move away from the midline of the body |
| **ad-** | toward, increasing | *adduct* means to move toward the midline of the body |
| **alb-** | white | *albino* is a person with a hereditary disorder *(albinism)* where there is partial or total absence of pigment in the skin |
| **ambi-** | both | *ambidextrous* is the ability to use both hands with equal dexterity |
| **ante-, pre-, pro-** | before | *antepartum* means before birth |
| **anti- contra-** | against | *antibiotic* means to act against microorganisms |
| **auto-** | self | *autologous* means relating to self |
| **bi- diplo-** | two | *bilateral* means pertaining to two sides |
| **bio-** | life | *biology* means the study of life |
| **brady-** | slow | *bradycardia* means a condition of slow heart rate |
| **con-** | together, with | *congenital* means present at birth |
| **circum-** | around | *circumcision* means the removal of the skin around the tip of the penis |
| **de-** | away from | *dehydration* is the process of water being taken away from the body |
| **dia-** | through | *diarrhea* is the rapid movement of fecal matter through the intestines |
| **dys-** | abnormal, difficult, painful | *dysuria* is painful urination |

(continued)

Table 6.1 Common Prefixes (continued)

| Prefixes | Meanings | Example |
|---|---|---|
| **ecto-** | outside | an *ectopic* pregnancy is when the ovum becomes fertilized outside the uterus |
| **endo-** | within | *endoscopy* is a procedure in which an instrument is placed within the body |
| **epi-** | upon, over | *epidermis* is the outermost layer of skin |
| **eu-** | normal, good | *eupepsia* is good digestion |
| **ex-, exo-, extra-** | out of, away from, outside | *exhale* means to breathe out |
| **hemi-, semi-** | half | *hemianosmia* is the absence of the sense of smell in one nostril; *semicircular* means shaped like a half-circle |
| **hyper-, poly-** | above normal, excessive | *hyperglycemia* is excess of glucose in the blood |
| **hypo-, sub-** | below normal, below, underneath | *hypoglycemia* is an abnormally low level of glucose in the blood |
| **inter-** | between | *intermuscular* means between muscles |
| **intra-** | within | *intradermal* means within the skin |
| **iso-** | same | *isotope* is a chemical element having the same atomic number as another chemical element |
| **macro-, megalo-** | big, large | *macromastia* is excessive breast size; *megalocephaly* is abnormally large head |
| **mal-** | bad, not adequate | *maldevelopment* is abnormal growth or development |
| **meta-** | change, transformation | *metastasis* is the transfer of disease from one organ to another organ not connected to it |
| **micro-** | small | *microscope* is an instrument used to enlarge an image of small objects such as cells |
| **mono-** | one | *monochromatic* means having only one color |
| **multi-, pluri-** | many | *multipara* is a term used to describe a woman who has had two or more pregnancies with viable offspring; also called *pluripara* |
| **neo-** | new, recent | *neonate* is a newborn |

(*continued*)

6 Medical Terminology

Table 6.1 Common Prefixes (concluded)

| Prefixes | Meanings | Example |
|---|---|---|
| **non-** | not | *noninvasive* is a term used to describe therapeutic and diagnostic procedures that do not involve the puncturing of the skin |
| **oligo-** | few, scanty, sparse | *oligomenorrhea* is scanty or infrequent menstruation |
| **pan-** | all | *pandemic* is a widespread epidemic, usually worldwide |
| **para-** | near, beside, beyond, opposite, abnormal | *parasomnia* is abnormal sleep patterns |
| **per-** | through | *percutaneous* means through the skin |
| **peri-** | around | *pericardium* is the fibrous sack around the heart |
| **poly-** | many | *polyarthritis* means arthritis of many joints |
| **post-** | after, following | *postmortem* means after death |
| **pre-** | before | *premature* means before maturation |
| **primi-** | first | *primipara* is a woman who has born one viable or living child |
| **quadra-, quadri-** | four | *quadriplegia* is paralysis of all four limbs |
| **re-** | again, backward | *relapse* is the return of a disease |
| **rube-** | red | *rubella* is a viral disease that produces red skin rashes |
| **semi-** | half | *semiconscious* means half conscious |
| **sub-** | under, below | *sublingual* means under the tongue |
| **super-, supra-** | above, superior | *supercilia* is the hair above the eye, otherwise known as eyebrows |
| **syn-, sym-** | together | *symbiosis* is mutual interdependence |
| **tachy-** | fast, abnormally fast | *tachycardia* is a fast heartbeat |
| **tri-** | three | *triceps* are muscles that have three heads |
| **ultra-** | beyond | *ultrasound* is a procedure where sound is used at very high frequency to study specific organs or organ systems |
| **uni-** | one, single | *unicellular* means made up of one cell |

## Table 6.2 Common Suffixes

| Suffixes | Meanings | Example |
|---|---|---|
| **-ac, -al, -ar, -ary** | pertaining to | *cardiac* is pertaining to the heart |
| **-algia** | pain | *gastralgia* means pain in the stomach |
| **-ase** | enzyme | *amylase* is a enzyme that breaks down food |
| **-blast** | baby, immature | *osteoblast* is an immature bone cell |
| **-cele** | abnormal protrusion | *rectocele* is an abnormal protrusion of the rectum into the vagina |
| **-centesis** | surgical puncture | *amniocentesis* is surgical puncture of the amniotic sac to obtain fluid |
| **-cide** | destroying | *germicide* is a solution that kills germs |
| **-cyte** | cell | *leukocyte* is a white blood cell |
| **-derma** | skin | *scleroderma* is the hardening of connective tissues |
| **-desis** | binding | *arthrodesis* is the binding of a joint |
| **-dynia** | pain | *gastrodynia* means pain in the stomach |
| **-ectomy** | surgical removal | *hysterectomy* is surgical removal of the uterus |
| **-edema** | fluid accumulation, swelling | *lymphedema* is chronic swelling in the lymph nodes usually due to an obstruction |
| **-emia** | blood | *anemia* is a low red blood cell condition |
| **-emesis** | vomiting | *hyperemesis* is excessive vomiting |
| **-esthesia** | sensation, feeling | *anesthesia* produces a lack of feeling |
| **-gen, -genesis** | producing, formation | *carcinogen* is something that produces cancer; *carcinogenesis* is the formation of the cancer |
| **-gram** | record | *electrocardiogram* is a recording of the variation of the heartbeat |
| **-graph** | instrument to record | *electrocardiograph* is the instrument used to record the heartbeat |
| **-iasis** | condition, formation of | *lithiasis* is the formation of stones |

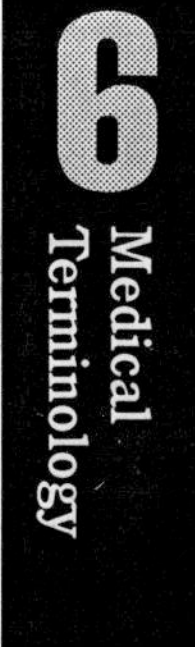


(continued)

Table 6.2 Common Suffixes (continued)

| Suffixes | Meanings | Example |
| --- | --- | --- |
| **-iatric** | pertaining to medical treatment | *pediatric* is pertaining to the medical treatment of children |
| **-ic, -ical** | pertaining to | *anemic* is pertaining to a patient who has anemia |
| **-ism** | condition | *hypothyroidism* is a condition of the thyroid gland |
| **-itis** | inflammation | *arthritis* is inflammation of a joint |
| **-logist** | someone who studies a specific area | *cardiologist* is a physician who studies the heart |
| **-logy** | the study of | *urology* is the study of the genitourinary tract |
| **-lysis** | destruction | *hemolysis* is the breaking down of blood |
| **-malacia** | softening | *encephalomalacia* is the softening of brain tissue |
| **-mania** | abnormal preoccupation | *megalomania* is a mental state characterized by delusions of personal importance or power |
| **-megaly** | enlargement | *cardiomegaly* is the enlargement of the heart |
| **-meter, -metry** | measuring device, the process of measuring | *spirometer* is a device for measuring airflow and volume of a person breathing |
| **-oma** | tumor | *carcinoma* is a cancerous malignant tumor |
| **-pathy** | disease | *idiopathy* is a disease of unknown origin |
| **-penia** | deficiency | *leukocytopenia* is the decrease in the number of white blood cells |
| **-pepsia** | digestion | *dyspepsia* is an upset stomach |
| **-pexy** | surgical fixation | *oophoropexy* means fixation or suspension of an ovary |
| **-phobia** | fear of | *acrophobia* is the fear of heights |

(continued)

Table 6.2 Common Suffixes (concluded)

| Suffixes | Meanings | Example |
|---|---|---|
| **-plasty** | surgical repair | *angioplasty* is the surgical repair of the blood vessels |
| **-pnea** | breath or breathing | *apnea* is the cessation of breathing |
| **-prandial** | meal | *postprandial* is after a meal |
| **-ptosis** | sagging or drooping | *hysteroptosis* is the prolapse of the uterus |
| **-rrhage, -rrhagia** | heavy discharge | *hemorrhage* is a heavy discharge of blood |
| **-rrhapy** | suturing | *ureterorrhaphy* is the suturing of the ureters |
| **-rrhea** | discharge | *amenorrhea* is the absence of menstrual flow |
| **-rrhexis** | rupture | *cardiorrhexis* is the rupture of the heart |
| **-scope** | an instrument | *microscope* is an instrument used to view very small objects |
| **-scopy** | process of using an instrument to assist in diagnosis or treatment | *microscopy* is the process of examining very small objects |
| **-stasis** | stopping | *hemostasis* is the stopping of the flow of blood |
| **-stenosis** | narrowing | *esophagostenosis* is the narrowing of the esophagus |
| **-stomy** | opening | *colostomy* is the creation of an opening between the colon and the surface of the body |
| **-tomy** | the process of cutting, an incision | *phlebotomy* is an incision into a vein |
| **-tropic** | nutrition | *atrophic* is a lack of nutrition |
| **-uria** | urine | *dysuria* is painful urination |

Every medical term has either a combining form or word root as part of the term. This is usually the main part of the medical term. A word root gives the medical term its central meaning. A combining form is where the word root is combined with a vowel to make the medical term easier to pronounce. The vowel used is usually an *o*, but may be an *i*.

The human body is divided into organ systems. We will look at each of those systems separately identifying the major word roots–combining forms in each system.

## Integumentary System

The *integumentary system* refers to the skin. It is the largest organ of the human body. The study of the skin is called dermatology. Most people will not recognize the term *integumentary* as referring to the skin.

The skin is composed of three layers: the epidermis or outer layer, the true skin or dermis, and the layer that anchors the skin called the hypodermis. *Hypo-* is a prefix that means below and *dermis* refers to skin.



Made up of not only our skin, but also the nails on our hands and feet, our hair, our sweat glands, oil glands, and some specialized glands, the skin is our first line of protection against infection. Our skin waterproofs our body and prevents fluid loss. Our skin helps the body synthesize vitamin D from the sun.

A dermatologist is a physician who specializes in diagnosing and treating diseases of the skin.

Table 6.3 lists common combining forms for the integumentary system.

## Musculoskeletal System

The *musculoskeletal system* is the structural support that is beneath the integumentary system. This system allows us to stand upright. The structure of the skeletal system includes bones, cartilage, ligaments, joints, and bursa. There are 206 bones in the human body. The body has more than 600 muscles that make up about 60% of the body's weight. Muscles are made up of fibers and are attached to bones by tendons. Ligaments are connective tissue that attaches bones to bones.

The skeletal system acts as a framework for the body and protects and supports the internal organs. The joints work in conjunction with muscles, tendons, and ligaments to allow for body movement. Our bones store calcium, which is necessary for nerve and muscle functions. Within the spongy part of the bones, red bone marrow is stored. Red bone marrow is important for the formation of blood cells.

Muscles hold our body erect and make movement possible. The movement of our muscles generates nearly 85% of the heat that keeps the body warm. Muscles move food through the digestive system. When we move our muscles, we are aiding the flow of blood through our veins as it returns to the heart.

## Table 6.3 Integumentary System

| Combining Forms | Meanings | Example |
|---|---|---|
| **adip/o** | fat | *adipose tissue* is the layer of fat beneath the skin |
| **albino/o** | white, without color | *albinism* is a condition that results in the lack of melanin pigment in the skin, eyes, and hair |
| **cry/o** | cold | *cryosurgery* is surgery that uses liquid nitrogen to freeze the tissue |
| **cutane/o** | skin | *subcutaneous* means beneath the skin |
| **cyan/o** | blue | *cyanosis* is a bluish discoloration of the skin |
| **dermat/o** | skin | *dermatitis* is an inflammation of the skin |
| **erythr/o, erythem/o** | red | *erythema* is redness of the skin caused by congestion of the capillaries |
| **hidr/o** | sweat | *hidropoiesis* is the formation of sweat |
| **hist/o** | tissue | *histology* is the study of tissues |
| **leuk/o** | white | *leucopenia* is a reduction of the number of leukocytes in the blood |
| **lip/o** | fat | *lipogenic* means anything that produces, forms, or is caused by fat |
| **melan/o** | black | *melanonychia* is the blackening of the nails by melanin pigmentation |
| **onych/o** | nail | *onychomalacia* is the softening of the nails |
| **scler/o** | hard, hardening | *scleroderma* is a condition of hardened skin |
| **seb/o** | sebum (oil) | *seborrhea* is a condition where there is excessive discharge from the sebaceous glands on the body |
| **trich/o** | hair | *trichoclasia* is brittle hair |
| **xanth/o** | yellow | *xanthoderma* is any yellow discoloration of the skin |
| **xer/o** | dry | *xeroderma* is excessive dryness of the skin |

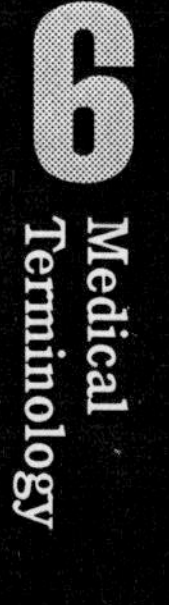

Several different medical specialists may be involved in the treatment of problems associated with the musculoskeletal system. An orthopedic surgeon specializes in diagnosing and treating the diseases and disorders associated with bones, joints, and muscles. A podiatrist holds a Doctor of Podiatric Medicine degree and specializes in diagnosing and treating disorders of the foot. Rheumatologists specialize in the diagnosis and treatment of rheumatic diseases that are characterized by inflammation in the connective tissues. A neurologist treats the cause of paralysis and similar muscular disorders in which there is a loss of function. A physiatrist is a physician who specializes in physical medicine and rehabilitation, and a sports medicine physician specializes in treating sports-related injuries of bones, muscles, and joints. Table 6.4 lists the most common combining forms for the musculoskeletal system.



**Table 6.4** Musculoskeletal System

| Combining Forms | Meanings | Example |
|---|---|---|
| **ankyl/o** | to make crooked; stiff | *ankylosis* is stiffness or immobility caused by disease or surgery |
| **arth/o** | joint | *arthritis* is inflammation of a joint |
| **carp/o** | wrist | *carpal tunnel syndrome* affects the nerves in the wrist |
| **cervic/o** | neck | *cervical* means pertaining to a neck |
| **chondr/o** | cartilage | *osteochondroma* is a benign cartilage and bone tumor |
| **cost/o** | rib | *intercostal* means between the ribs |
| **cran/o** | skull, head | *craniomalacia* means softening of the skull |
| **dors/o** | back | *dorsal* is toward the back |
| **kyph/o** | hump | *kyphosis* is abnormal curvature of the spine |
| **lamin/o** | thin flat plate or layer of a vertebra | *laminectomy* is the surgical removal of the lamina |

(*continued*)

Table 6.4 Musculoskeletal System (concluded)

| Combining Forms | Meanings | Example |
|---|---|---|
| **lei/o** | smooth muscle | *leiomyoma* is a benign tumor of the smooth muscle |
| **myo, /myos/o** | muscle | *myalgia* is muscle pain; *myositis* is the inflammation of muscle tissue |
| **orth/o** | straight | *orthopedist* is a surgeon who specializes in straightening bones |
| **oste/o** | bone | *osteitis* in inflammation of the bone |
| **ten/o** | tendon | *tendonitis* means inflammation of a tendon |



## Cardiovascular System

The *cardiovascular system* pertains to the heart (cardio) and the blood vessels (vascular). The cardiovascular structures work together to pump blood to all of our body tissues. Blood moves cellular waste products to various organs for removal from the body and also supplies oxygen and nutrients to tissues throughout the body. Blood cells play an important role in both the immune and endocrine systems.

Hematologists specialize in diagnosing and treating diseases and disorders related to the blood and blood-forming tissues. Cardiologists specialize in diagnosing and treating abnormalities, diseases, and disorders of the heart. There are several types of cardiologists who specialize in specific areas of cardiology. A pediatric cardiologist has special training in treating and preventing heart and blood vessel disease in infants, children, and teenagers. A cardiac surgeon has special training to perform delicate operations on the heart and associated organs.

The main terms for the cardiovascular system are found in Table 6.5.

## Respiratory System

The *respiratory system* is our breathing system. By bringing oxygen into the body for the blood cells, the respiratory system performs a vital service. The respiratory system also expels carbon dioxide and other waste when we breathe out. Airflow through the larynx makes talking possible. The organs in the respiratory system include the nose, tonsils, paranasal sinuses, pharynx, epiglottis, larynx, trachea, lungs, and diaphragm.

Table 6.5 Cardiovascular System

| Combining Forms | Meanings | Example |
|---|---|---|
| **angi/o** | vessel | *angiospasm* is the spasmodic contraction of the walls of a blood vessel |
| **aort/o** | aorta | *aortostenosis* is the narrowing of the aorta |
| **arteri/o** | artery | *arteriosclerosis* is the thickening of an arterial wall |
| **atri/o** | atrium | *atriomegaly* is the abnormal enlargement of the atrium |
| **cardi/o** | heart | *cardiologist* is a physician who specializes in treatment of heart diseases |
| **cyt/o** | cell | *cytology* is the study of the cell |
| **erythr/o** | red | *erythrocytes* are red blood cells |
| **hem/o** | blood | *hemorrhage* is the abnormal discharge of blood |
| **leuk/o** | white | *leukemia* is a malignancy characterized by an increase in the number of abnormal white blood cells |
| **lymph/o** | lymph | *lymphangioma* is a benign tumor formed by an abnormal collection of lymphatic vessels |
| **phleb/o** | vein | *phlebotomist* is a technician who draws blood |
| **plasm/o** | plasma | *plasmapheresis* is the removal of plasma from the body |
| **thromb/o** | clot | *thrombophlebitis* is an inflammation of the vein |
| **valv/o** | valve | *valvular prolapse* is an abnormal protrusion of a heart value |
| **vas/o** | vessel | *vasoconstrictor* is a medication that constricts the blood vessels |
| **ven/o** | vein | *venipuncture* is the puncture of a vein for the purpose of drawing blood |
| **ventricul/o** | ventricular | *ventriculopuncture* is the surgical puncture of the lateral ventricle of the brain |

An otolaryngologist specializes in diagnosing and treating diseases and disorders of the ear, nose, and throat. This specialty is often referred to as ENT for ear, nose, and throat. A pulmonologist specializes in diagnosing and treating diseases and disorders of the lungs. Some of the common combining forms for the respiratory system may be found in Table 6.6.

**Table 6.6** Respiratory System

| Combining Forms | Meanings | Example |
|---|---|---|
| **aer/o** | air | *aerophagia* is the excessive swallowing of air |
| **alveol/o** | air sac | *alveoalgia* is pain in the *alveolus* of a tooth after extraction |
| **bronch/o** | bronchus or bronchi | *bronchitis* is the inflammation of the bronchi in the upper respiratory tract |
| **laryng/o** | larynx | *laryngitis* is the inflammation of the mucous membrane of the larynx |
| **lob/o** | lobes | *lobectomy* is the surgical excision of a lobe—in the lung, brain, liver, or thyroid |
| **muc/o** | mucus | *mucolytic* is an agent that destroys mucus |
| **nas/o, rhin/o** | nose | *nasal* sprays are used to relieve symptoms of rhinitis |
| **ox/o** | oxygen | *hypoxia* is deficiency of oxygen in tissues |
| **pleur/o** | pleura | *pleurisy* is an inflammation of the pleura around one of the lungs |
| **pneum/o** | lung, air | *pneumonia* is an inflammation of the lung |
| **pulmon/o** | lung | *pulmonary* edema is extravascular fluid in lung tissue usually from left ventricular failure |
| **sinus/o** | sinus | *sinusitis* is the inflammation of the lining of the paranasal sinuses |
| **spir/o** | to breathe | *spirometry* is the making of airflow and volume measurements with a spirometer |
| **tonsil/o** | tonsils | *tonsillectomy* is the removal of the tonsils |
| **trache/o** | trachea | *tracheotomy* is the operation done to create an opening in the trachea; this is usually intended to be temporary |

## Gastrointestinal System

The *gastrointestinal (GI) system* is responsible for the intake and digestion of food. The GI system is also responsible for absorbing nutrients from the digested food, as well as the elimination of solid waste products in our bodies. The GI tract consists of the mouth, esophagus, and stomach (the upper GI tract) as well as the small and large intestines, rectum, and anus (the lower GI tract). Other organs that are also an important part of the GI system include the liver, gallbladder, and pancreas. Table 6.7 lists the major combining forms used in the GI system.



### Table 6.7 Gastrointestinal System

| Combining Forms | Meanings | Example |
|---|---|---|
| **ailment/o** | nourishment or food | *alimentary* canal is another name for the digestive tract |
| **amyl/o** | starch | *amylorrhea* is the passage of undigested starch in the stools |
| **bil/i** | bile | *biliary* cirrhosis is a liver disorder due to the obstruction of bile ducts |
| **chol/e** | gall, bile | *cholangiography* is the radiographic examination of the bile ducts |
| **cholecyst/o** | gallbladder | *cholecystotomy* is a surgical incision into the gallbladder |
| **col/o** | colon | *colonoscopy* is the visual examination of the colon |
| **cyst/o** | bladder | *cystalgia* is pain in the urinary bladder |
| **dent/o** | tooth | *dentalgia* is a toothache |
| **duoden/o** | duodenum | *duodenorrhaphy* is the suture of a tear or incision in the duodenum |
| **enter/o** | intestine | *enteritis* is the inflammation of the small intestine |
| **esophag/o** | esophagus | *esophagogastroduodenoscopy* (EGD) is the endoscopic examination of the esophagus, stomach, and duodenum |
| **gastr/o** | stomach | *gastroesophageal* reflux disease (GERD) is a syndrome of chronic epigastric pain, accompanied by belching and nausea |

(continued)

Table 6.7 Gastrointestinal System (concluded)

| Combining Forms | Meanings | Example |
|---|---|---|
| **gingiv/o** | gums | *gingivitis* is the inflammation of the gums |
| **gloss/o** | tongue | *glossodynia* is a condition characterized by a burning or painful tongue |
| **hepat/o** | liver | *hepatitis* is an inflammation of the liver usually from a viral infection |
| **intest/o** | intestines | *intestinal* villi are the projections of mucous membranes in the intestine |
| **lapar/o** | abdomen | *laparoscope* is an endoscope used for examining the peritoneal cavity |
| **lip/o** | fat | *lipedema* is painful swelling of subcutaneous fat, especially in the legs of women |
| **lith/o** | stone | *lithotripsy* is the crushing of a stone in the renal pelvis, ureter, or bladder by either sound waves or mechanical force |
| **or/o** | mouth | *orally* is by or through the mouth |
| **pancreat/o** | pancreas | *pancreatolithiasis* is a condition in which there are stones in the pancreas or pancreatic duct system |
| **peritone/o** | peritoneum | *peritoneum* is the serous membrane that lines the abdominal cavity |
| **phag/o** | eat | *phagocyte* is a cell that ingests bacteria, foreign particles, and other cells |
| **pharyng/o** | pharynx | *pharyngitis* is the inflammation of the pharynx |
| **proct/o** | rectum | *proctoscopy* is the visual examination of the rectum and anus with a proctoscope |
| **rect/o** | rectum | *rectal* means relating to the rectum |
| **sigmoid/o** | sigmoid colon | *sigmoidopexy* is a surgical procedure to attach the sigmoid colon to a firm structure to correct rectal prolapse |
| **stomat/o** | mouth | *stomatomalacia* is the pathologic softening of any structures in the mouth |

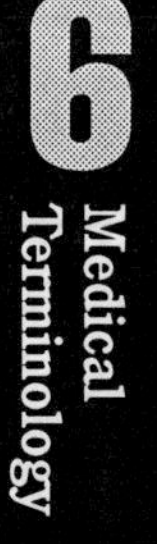

## Urinary System

The *urinary system* is made up of the two kidneys, two ureters, one bladder, and the urethra. The urinary system is important in maintaining the proper balance of water, salts, and acids in the body fluids by removing excess fluids from the body. Constantly filtering the blood to remove urea (the major waste product of protein metabolism), the urinary system also removes other waste products from the bloodstream. The waste products and excess fluids are converted into urine and excreted through the urinary bladder. All of these functions are important in maintaining homeostasis which is the state of equilibrium that produces a constant internal environment throughout the body.

The physician who diagnoses and treats diseases and disorders of the urinary system is called a urologist. A nephrologist specializes in diagnosing and treating diseases of the kidneys.

The major combining forms for the urinary system are contained in Table 6.8.



## Nervous System

The *nervous system* is responsible for coordinating and controlling all bodily activities. The brain is the center of the nervous system. Other structures in the nervous system include the nerves, the spinal cord, and the sensory organs and receptors (eyes, ears, nose, skin, and

**Table 6.8** Urinary System

| Combining Forms | Meanings | Example |
|---|---|---|
| **albumin/o** | protein, albumin | *albuminuria* refers to albumin in the urine |
| **bacteri/o** | bacteria | *bacteriuria* is bacteria in the urine |
| **cyst/o** | urinary bladder | *cystitis* is inflammation of the urinary bladder |
| **lith/o** | stone | *nephrolithiasis* is the presence of a kidney stone |
| **nephr/o** | kidney | *nephrectomy* is the removal of the kidney |
| **olig/o** | few; scanty | *oliguria* is scanty urine production |
| **pyel/o** | renal pelvis | *pyelolithotomy* is the surgical removal of stones from the renal pelvis |
| **ren/i, ren/o** | kidney | *renography* is radiography of the kidney |
| **ur/o** | urine | *urinalysis* is the analysis of the urine to help diagnose diseases |

tongue). The sensory organs are for our five senses: sight, hearing, smell, touch, and taste. Terms for the nose, skin, and tongue were covered earlier in the discussion of the gastrointestinal and integumentary systems. The eyes and the ears will be covered separately.

The nervous system is divided into two primary parts. The first part is the central nervous system which is the brain and spinal cord. The peripheral nervous system contains the 12 pairs of cranial nerves extending from the brain, as well as the 31 pairs of spinal nerves that extend from the spinal cord.

There are several different medical specialties that treat various aspects of the nervous system. An anesthesiologist specializes in administering anesthesia before and during surgery. A neurologist specializes in diagnosing and treating diseases and disorders of the nervous system. A neurosurgeon specializes in surgery of the nervous system. A psychiatrist specializes in diagnosing and treating disorders of the mind such as chemical dependency, mental illness, and emotional problems. A psychologist has earned an advanced degree in psychology and is not a medical doctor, as are the previously mentioned specialists, but is licensed to treat emotional problems and mental illness.

The combining forms associated with the nervous system are found in Table 6.9.



**Table 6.9** Nervous System

| Combining Forms | Meanings | Example |
|---|---|---|
| **cerebr/o** | cerebrum | *cerebral palsy* is a motor disorder caused by damage to the brain |
| **encephal/o** | brain | *encephalitis* is the inflammation of the brain |
| **mening/o** | the membranes covering the brain and spinal cord | *meningoencephalitis* is the inflammation of the brain and the meninges |
| **myel/o** | spinal cord | *myelography* is the radiography of the spinal cord after an injection of a contrast dye |
| **neur/o** | nerve | *neuroma* is a tumor or growth made up of nerve cells and nerve fibers |
| **psych/o** | mind | *psychometry* is the testing and measuring of mental and psychological ability |

## Endocrine System

The primary function of the *endocrine system* is to produce hormones. Hormones are chemical transmitters with a specific regulatory effect. Hormones are secreted directly into the bloodstream, allowing them to reach cells and organs throughout the body. There are 13 major glands in the endocrine system. A gland is a ductless organ that secretes the hormones and releases them directly into circulation. These glands are the pituitary gland, thyroid gland, four parathyroid glands, two adrenal glands, one pancreas, one thymus, one pineal gland, and two gonads (ovaries in females and testes in males). The endocrine and the nervous system are the two major control systems of the body and their functions are interrelated.



The physician that diagnoses and treats diseases and disorders of the endocrine system is called an endocrinologist. The combining forms for the endocrine system are found in Table 6.10.

## Reproductive Systems

The primary function of the *female reproductive system* is to create and support new life. Mature eggs are produced by the ovaries and are fertilized by male sperm. The uterus provides the environment and support for the developing child. The female breast produces

**Table 6.10** Endocrine System

| Combining Forms | Meanings | Example |
|---|---|---|
| **aden/o** | gland | *adenosis* is any disease of a gland |
| **andr/o** | male | *androgen* is a hormone produced in the testes in males |
| **adrenal/o** | adrenal gland | *adrenalectomy* is the surgical removal of one or both of the adrenal glands |
| **cortic/o** | cortex | *corticosteroid* is a steroid produced by the adrenal cortex |
| **gluc/o** | sugar | *glucosuria* is sugar in the urine |
| **gonad/o** | sex gland | *gonadopathy* is any disease of the gonads |
| **thym/o** | thymus gland | *thymoma* is a tumor made up of epithelial or lymphoid elements of the thymus |
| **thry/o** | thyroid gland | *thyroaplasia* is the defective development of the thyroid with deficient activity of its secretions |

milk for the new child. The major organs of the female reproductive system are the vagina, uterus, fallopian tubes, ovaries, mammary glands, and ducts.

The primary function of the *male reproductive system* is to produce sperm and deliver them into the female body. Some of the structures of the male reproductive system also function as part of the urinary system. The major organs of the male reproductive system are the testicles, penis, scrotum, vas deferens, and prostate gland.

Physicians who treat and diagnose diseases of the female reproductive system are called gynecologists. If the physician also delivers babies, he or she is an obstetrician-gynecologist. Urologists treat not only urinary system problems in males and females, but also diseases and disorders of the genitourinary system in males. The major combining forms for the reproductive systems are found in Table 6.11.



### Table 6.11 Reproductive Systems

| Combining Forms | Meanings | Example |
|---|---|---|
| **amni/o** | amnion | *amniocentesis* is a surgical puncture of the amnion for diagnostic testing |
| **cervic/o** | cervix | *cervicitis* is the inflammation of the cervix uteri |
| **colp/o** | vagina | *colposcopy* is an examination of the vagina with a lighted instrument |
| **crypt/o** | concealed | *cryptorchidism* is when the testes do not descend in fetal development |
| **gon/o** | genitals | *gonorrhea* is the highly contagious bacterial infection of the genitourinary system |
| **gyn/o** | woman, female | *gynecomastia* is the excessive development of mammary glands in the male |
| **hyster/o** | uterus | *hysterectomy* is surgical removal of the uterus |
| **mamm/o, mast/o** | breast | *mammalgia* and *mastalgia* both mean pain in the breast |
| **meno/o** | menstruation | *amenorrhea* is absence of menstruation |
| **nat/o** | birth | *neonatal* is the first month of life |
| **oophor/o** | ovary | *oophorocystectomy* is the removal of an ovarian cyst |
| **orchid/o** | testes, testicle | *orchiectomy* is the removal of one or both testes |
| **salping/o** | fallopian tube | *bilateral salpingo-oophorectomy* is the excision of both fallopian tubes and ovaries |
| **vas/o** | vessel, duct | *vasectomy* is the removal of a section of the vas deferens |

## Special Senses—Eyes and Ears

Our eyes are the receptor organs of vision. The functions of the eyes are to receive images and transmit them to the brain. The extraocular (outside the eyeball) structures are the orbit or socket, six muscles, eyelids, eyebrows and eyelashes, conjunctiva, and the lacrimal apparatus. Conjunctiva is the mucous membrane that lines the underside of each eyelid. The lacrimal apparatus is the structure that produces, stores, and removes tears. The intraocular structures are the eyeball; the sclera and cornea; the uveal tract made up of the iris, pupil, and lens; and the retina.

Ophthalmologists are medical doctors who treat eye and vision diseases and disorders. Optometrists hold a Doctor of Optometry degree. They specialize in measuring the vision in our eyes to determine if corrective lenses are necessary. The combining forms for the eye are found in Table 6.12.

The ears are the receptor organs of hearing. The functions of the ears are to receive sound and transmit those sounds to the brain. The inner ear also plays a part in maintaining our balance. The outer ear structures are the pinna or auricle, the external auditory canal. It is cerumen or earwax that is secreted by glands in the auditory canal. The middle



**Table 6.12** The Eye

| Combining Forms | Meanings | Example |
|---|---|---|
| **blephar/o** | eyelid | *blepharitis* is the inflammation of the eyelids |
| **conjunctiv/o** | conjunctiva | *conjunctivitis* is the inflammation of the conjunctiva, better known as pinkeye |
| **dacry/o** | tear duct | *dacryorrhea* is the excessive flow of tears |
| **dipl/o** | double | *diplopia* is the perception of two images of one object, better known as double vision |
| **nyct/o** | night | *nyctalopia* is poor night vision |
| **ocul/o** | eye | *oculomycosis* is any fungal disease of the eye |
| **phot/o** | light | *photoretinitis* is retinitis due to exposure to intense light |
| **presby/o** | old | *presbyopia* is the loss of vision with old age |

Table 6.13 The Ear

| Combining Forms | Meanings | Example |
|---|---|---|
| **acous/o** | hearing | *acoustic* is pertaining to hearing |
| **audi/o** | hearing | *audiometer* is an instrument to measure hearing |
| **myring/o** | tympanic membrane | *myringectomy* is the excision of the tympanic membrane |
| **ot/o** | ear | *otitis media* is the inflammation of the middle ear |
| **tympan/o** | tympanic membrane | *tympanoplasty* is the surgical fixation of the tympanic membrane after perforation |



ear contains the tympanic membrane or eardrum, as well as three small bones called the malleus (the hammer), the incus (the anvil), and the stapes (the stirrup). The inner ear contains the sensory receptors for hearing and balance: the cochlea, vestibule, and semicircular canals.

An audiologist specializes in measuring of hearing function and in the rehabilitation of people with hearing impairments. The main combining forms for the ears are found in Table 6.13.

## Abbreviations

Abbreviations are used throughout the health care community. Most are in common usage. Some offices set up their own particular abbreviations. The most commonly used abbreviations may be found in Table 6.14. Abbreviations must be used with caution, however, as they may mean different things to different people. For example, *MS* may mean musculoskeletal, multiple sclerosis, morphine sulfate, or magnesium sulfate. *MS* is on the "do not use" list published by the Joint Commission on Accreditation of Healthcare Organizations (JCAHO). This list appears in Table 6.15.

**Table 6.14** Commonly Used Medical Abbreviations

| Abbreviations | Meanings |
|---|---|
| AMA | against medical advice |
| ASHD | arteriosclerotic heart disease |
| BP | blood pressure |
| bpm | beats per minute |
| C | Celsius, centigrade |
| CA, ca | cancer |
| CBC | complete blood count |
| CC | chief complaint |
| CCU | coronary care unit |
| CNS | central nervous system |
| C/O | complains of |
| CP | chest pain |
| CPE | complete physical exam |
| COPD | chronic obstructive pulmonary disease |
| CVA | cerebrovascular accident (stroke) |
| D&C | dilation and curettage |
| DX | diagnosis |
| ECG, EKG | electrocardiogram |
| EEG | electroencephalogram |
| EGD | esophagogastroduodenoscopy |
| F | Fahrenheit |
| FH | family history |
| FL | fluid |
| GERD | gastroesophageal reflux disease |
| GI | gastrointestinal |
| GU | genitourinary |
| GYN | gynecology |
| H&P | history and physical |
| HEENT | head, hears, eyes, nose, and throat |
| HT | height |
| HX | history |
| I&D | incision and drainage |
| ICU | intensive care unit |

(*continued*)

**Table 6.14** Commonly Used Medical Abbreviations (concluded)

| Abbreviations | Meanings |
|---|---|
| IP | inpatient |
| IV | intravenous |
| MI | myocardial infarction |
| N&V | nausea and vomiting |
| OP | outpatient |
| OPD | outpatient department |
| OR | operating room |
| P | pulse |
| PAR | postanesthetic recovery |
| PE | physical exam |
| PI | present illness |
| PMH | past medical history |
| POSTOP | postoperative |
| P&P | pap smear and pelvic exam |
| PREOP | preoperative |
| PT | patient |
| R/O | rule out |
| RE✓ | recheck |
| REF | referral |
| ROS/SR | review of systems/systems review |
| Rx | prescription |
| SOB | shortness of breath |
| T | temperature |
| TPR | temperature, pulse, and respirations |
| TX, TR | treatment |
| UA | urinalysis |
| UCHD | usual childhood diseases |
| UGI | upper GI |
| URI | upper respiratory infection |
| US | ultrasound |
| UTI | urinary tract infection |
| VS | vital signs |
| WDWN | well developed, well nourished |
| WNL | within normal limits |
| WT | weight |
| YO | year old |

## Table 6.15 JCAHO's Do Not Use List

| Official "Do Not Use" List* | | |
|---|---|---|
| **Do Not Use** | **Potential Problem** | **Use Instead** |
| U (unit) | Mistaken for "0" (zero), the number "4" (four) or "cc" | Write "unit" |
| IU (International Unit) | Mistaken for IV (intravenous) or the number 10 (ten) | Write "International Unit" |
| Q.D., QD, q.d., qd (daily) | Mistaken for each other | Write "daily" |
| Q.O.D., QOD, q.o.d. qod (every other day) | Period after the Q mistaken for "I" and the "O" mistaken for "I" | Write "every other day" |
| Trailing zero (X.0 mg)† Lack of leading zero (.X mg) | Decimal point is missed | Write X mg Write 0.X mg |
| MS | Can mean morphine sulfate or magnesium sulfate | Write "morphine sulfate" |
| $MSO_4$ and $MgSO_4$ | Confused for one another | Write "magnesium sulfate" |

*Applies to all orders and all medication-related documentation that is handwritten (including free-text computer entry) or on preprinted forms

†**Exception:** A "trailing zero" may be used only where required to demonstrate the level of precision of the value being reported, such as for laboratory results, imaging studies that report size of lesions, or catheter/tube sizes. It may not be used in medication orders or other medication-related documentation.

*(continued)*

**Table 6.15** JCAHO's Do Not Use List (concluded)

| Additional Abbreviations, Acronyms and Symbols (For *possible* future inclusion in the Official "Do Not Use" List) | | |
|---|---|---|
| **Do Not Use** | **Potential Problem** | **Use Instead** |
| > (greater than)<br>< (less than) | Misinterpreted as the number "7" (seven) or the letter "L"<br>Confused for one another | Write "greater than"<br>Write "less than" |
| Abbreviations for drug names | Misinterpreted due to similar abbreviations for multiple drugs | Write drug names in full |
| Apothecary units | Unfamiliar to many practitioners<br>Confused with metric units | Use metric units |
| @ | Mistaken for the number "2" (two) | Write "at" |
| cc | Mistaken for U (units) when poorly written | Write "ml" or "milliliters" |
| µg | Mistaken for mg (milligrams) resulting in one thousand-fold overdose | Write "mcg" or "micrograms" |

Source: © The Joint Commission, 2008. Reprinted with permission.

## Measurements

In medicine, measurements are based on the metric system. Metric units include the meter, gram, and liter. The meter (m) equals 39.37 inches and is used for length. The liter (L or l) is used for volume and 1 liter equals approximately 1.056 U.S. quarts. The gram (g or gm) is used for weight and it is equal to 0.035 ounce. Table 6.16 lists the common abbreviations found in the metric system.



**Table 6.16** Metric System Abbreviations

| Abbreviations | Meaning |
|---|---|
| cc | cubic centimeter (1 cc = 1 mL) |
| cm | centimeter (2.54 cm = 1 inch) |
| g or gm | gram |
| kg | kilogram (1 kg = 1000 gm = 2.2 lb) |
| km | kilometer |
| L or l | liter = 1,000 mL (1 gallon = 4 quarts = 8 pints = 3.785 L; 1 pint = 473.17 mL) |
| mL | milliliter |
| mm | millimeter |

## Summary

Learning medical terminology is important for your success in the medical office. You are probably already familiar with many medical terms. Be sure you learn the meaning of those terms that are specific to your office. Remember that many medical terms are made up of interchangeable word parts that are used in different combinations to form the word. Also remember that there may be more than one word that means the same thing. Become comfortable with the words so that you have a better understanding of what is happening in your office.

# Chapter 7

# Medical Records and Privacy

**Introduction** *In any business, records must be kept. In the medical office, the medical record or chart is the most important record that is kept. The medical record serves a variety of purposes for the practice. The importance of an accurate medical record cannot be overstated. All medical records are considered private, and maintaining that privacy is critical for all staff members to keep in mind.*

## Chapter Outline

## Why Do We Keep Medical Records?

First, the medical record documents the course of medical treatment of the patient. It provides information about the management and evaluation of the patient's care. The record charts the changes in the patient's condition and documents any need for further follow-up.

Second, the medical record documents communication between the members of the practice and the patient, as well as communication between the providers in the practice and other health care providers. The medical record often contains reports from other providers and laboratories, as well as radiology (X-ray) and diagnostic reports.

The medical record serves as a foundation for the planning of a patient's care and continuity in the evaluation of the care. Not only is the patient's history contained in a medical record, so is the family history as well as the other medical reports already mentioned.

Fourth, the medical record serves as legal documentation of the care provided to the patient. The importance of accurate and complete medical records cannot be overemphasized.

Last, for both database purposes and chart audits done by insurance companies, a complete and accurate medical record is necessary. Accurate medical records are important in continuing education and research. Insurance companies look for documentation of care on a routine basis.



## What Is in a Medical Record?

Although every medical practice may organize the medical record in a slightly different way, there are certain items that may be contained in every medical record. Table 7.1 lists the major information usually found in a medical record.

In a paper medical record, the information is standardized for each chart. Although practices vary, usually the right-hand side of the chart contains the clinical information beginning with the patient's first visit, and the left-hand side contains the rest of the information. Dividers of some type are often used to further organize the information.

In today's electronic environment, use of the **electronic medical record (EMR)** or **electronic health record (EHR)** is growing. The EMR is covered in more detail in Chapter 4. Much of the patient's information comes to the practice in an electronic fashion, but there is still a lot of paper to put in a chart. Many practices are already using EMRs. Eventually, it is anticipated that all health care records will move to the electronic environment, but as outlined in Chapter 4, there are many complications involved in getting all practices to use EMR.

**Table 7.1** Major Information Found in a Medical Record

- Demographic information and authorizations
- Medical history from the patient
- Past medical records from other health care providers
- Insurance and financial information
- Progress notes
- Diagnostic test results, lab and X-ray results, and other clinical data (hospitalizations, therapy treatments, reports from other physicians about current treatments)
- Medications
- Correspondence
- Referrals

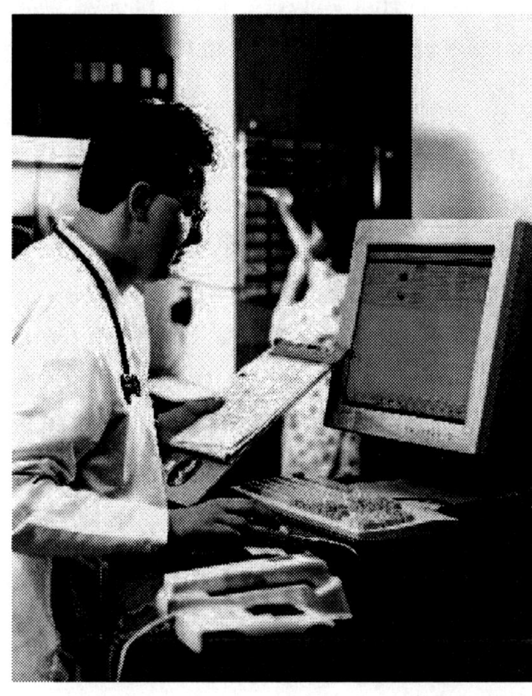

Use of the electronic medical record is increasing.

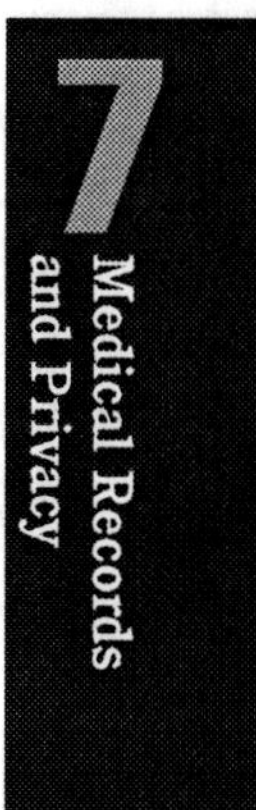

## Demographic Information and Authorizations

Every patient completes a registration or patient data sheet. A sample registration form is found in Chapter 10. The form usually contains an authorization to release medical records to insurance companies and other third-party payers. However, in order for a patient's medical record to be released to other physicians, therapists, and care providers, a separate authorization must be completed. A sample form is found later in this chapter (Figure 7.3).

Most practices have the patient fill out a patient and family history form. This form varies from practice to practice. Specific types of practices may ask for very specific information beyond the general health history. Specialty practices may add information pertinent to their specialty.

## Past Medical Records from Other Health Care Providers

Many times patients bring a copy of their past medical records from other providers. Also, there is often a need to request medical records from other providers in order to give the provider a clearer picture of the patient's problems. These records are not the property of the new treating provider and cannot be released to anyone by the new provider. If the patient requests that the records be placed in his or her chart, make a copy and place them in the chart, returning the records to the patient. Be sure to note in the chart that you returned the copy to the patient. Further discussion about release of information can be found later in the chapter.



## Insurance and Financial Information

In Chapter 8 the importance of collecting current information is discussed. It is also important to advise the patient of the practice's financial policies. Many times patients assume certain things that are incorrect. For example, if an insurance company denies payment for any reason, that does not mean the patient does not owe the charges for the services rendered. Also, patients often don't understand the meaning of deductible, copayment, and coinsurance, so it is important to have a written financial policy for the patients to read. Have patients sign an acknowledgment that they received the financial policies. A sample financial policy statement is found in Chapter 10.

## Progress Notes

The chronological listing of all patient visits, prescription refills, calls from the patient, and calls pertinent to the patient is called the progress notes. The fundamental rule is that anytime a patient has an interaction with anyone in the practice, it should be recorded in the patient's progress notes.

Progress notes are arranged in chronological order, with the most recent date on top. Usually, several notes are recorded on one page so the latest note should be the last one on the page. Every practice will have guidelines about how to document information and what, if any, abbreviations are acceptable. Again, be cautious when using abbreviations. In Chapter 6 you will find some of the JCAHO restrictions on abbreviations, as well as a detailed list of acceptable abbreviations.

Progress notes are often documented in a format using the SOAP method. The SOAP method used consistently helps all providers form a clearer picture of the patient's condition. It works particularly well in multispecialty group practices because it allows for continuity of care. This method, as well as HPIP, provides for consistent information in the same place in the patient's record. Here is how they differ:

SOAP

- S—subjective information
- O—objective clinical evidence
- A—assessment or diagnosis
- P—plans for further studies, treatment, or management

HPIP

- H—history (subjective information)
- P—physical exam (objective clinical information)
- I—impression (assessment/diagnosis)
- P—plan (treatment)

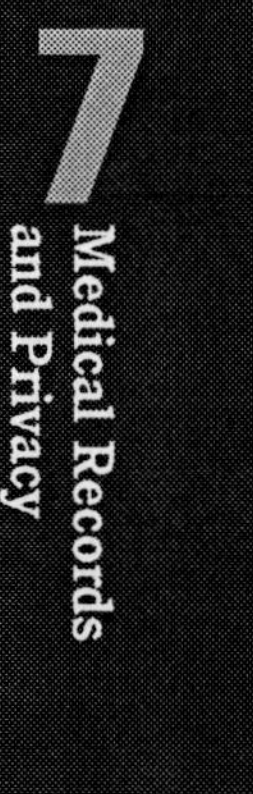


## Diagnostic Test Results, Lab and X-Ray Results, and Other Clinical Data

The amount of other health information included in a patient's medical record depends on the type of practice, the patient's medical condition, and the reasons the patient is being treated. Some practices separate the types of information in the report. For example, X-ray results may be filed separately from lab results or other clinical data, depending on the type of practice. It is important, however, that the other clinical data are sorted in chronological order with the most recent information on top.

## Medications

Within the progress notes, the medications prescribed are documented. However, in order for the provider to have a clearer clinical picture, a separate medication list is often used as part of the medical record. It is often combined with some other items in a problem-based list. Figure 7.1 illustrates a sample problem list. Individual practices may add items to this one-page sheet, depending on the specialty.

## Problem and Medication List

Patient Name: ________________ DOB: ______________

Allergies:

| |
|---|
| ______________________________ |
| ______________________________ |
| ______________________________ |

Pharmacy: ________________ Phone# ________________

| DATE: | Rx / Refill |
|---|---|
| Start:___ Stop:___ | ___ Initials |
| Start:___ Stop:___ | ___ Initials |
| Start:___ Stop:___ | ___ Initials |
| Start:___ Stop:___ | ___ Initials |
| Start:___ Stop:___ | ___ Initials |
| Start:___ Stop:___ | ___ Initials |
| Start:___ Stop:___ | ___ Initials |
| Start:___ Stop:___ | ___ Initials |
| Start:___ Stop:___ | ___ Initials |
| Start:___ Stop:___ | ___ Initials |
| | ___ |
| | ___ |

Chronic Problems:

| Date: | Problem / Medication |
|---|---|
| | |
| | |
| | |
| | |
| | |
| | |
| | |
| | |
| | |
| | |

Figure 7.1 Problem List

### Correspondence

This part of the medical record could include all letters and other correspondence regarding the patient. Some practices put only nonclinical information in this section, but other practices include letters from other physicians regarding the patient's treatment. It is recommended that the correspondence section include only nonclinical information to avoid the possibility that important clinical information is overlooked by clinical personnel.

### Referrals

Many health insurance plans require that providers follow very specific rules when referring patients to specialists. There is often a specific form that must be completed. These completed forms would be found in the referral section. Often practices file this information under correspondence.

## Privacy, the Medical Record, and HIPAA

A basic principle that has always existed to a certain degree is that a patient's medical record is private information to be shared only with the patient and the health care provider(s) involved in the patient's care. Although usually for good reason, in the past this principle was not always enforced. As our country became more privacy focused, a variety of laws have been passed. The major federal law that governs privacy is the **Health Insurance Portability and Accountability Act of 1996 (HIPAA).** This law required several changes for everyone in the health care industry.

Many people believe that HIPAA is concerned only with the privacy of the patient's medical record. HIPAA actually covers much more. *Portability* refers to an individual's right to portability in his or her health insurance. Before HIPAA, preexisting conditions were not necessarily covered as an individual moved from one group plan to another. This made changing jobs difficult if you had any health conditions. Employers sought legislative help to fix this problem. Part of the HIPAA legislation corrected the problem of preexisting conditions when moving from one group health insurance to another group health insurance. That does not necessarily mean that all preexisting conditions are automatically covered. If the new plan does not cover the condition to start with, the plan will not cover the condition for the individual employee.

The *accountability* portion of HIPAA has four standards. Each one has had a dramatic impact on how the business of health care is conducted. The standards cover transactions and code sets, privacy, security, and a national identifier number (NPI). Table 7.2 provides an explanation of those standards.

Table 7.2 HIPAA Standards

| HIPAA Standard Number | Purpose |
|---|---|
| Standard #1 Transactions and Code Sets | This standard was designed to bring uniformity and simplification to the billing and coding of health care services. By requiring the use of standard formats and data content when transmitting files electronically, the billing and payment process should be easier and more efficient. |
| Standard #2 Privacy Rule | Protecting the privacy of patient-identifying information is the primary purpose of this standard. Patients were given additional rights under this standard. |
| Standard #3 Security Rule | Electronically transmitted protected health information (PHI) must be transmitted in a secure manner by using firewalls, antivirus software, encryption and password protection, as well as other security measures. |
| Standard #4 National Identifier | Requires a standard single identifier for providers, health plans, employers, and individuals. |



Standard #2, the privacy rule, is designed to protect the privacy of individually identifiable health information. It took effect April 14, 2003, after much public and industry discussion. The standard sets forth a list of covered entities required to protect the privacy of the patient and the patient's record. Much of the standard pertains to electronic transmittal, but all medical records are covered.

The new standard gives patients new rights to access their medical records and to restrict access by others. Patients have the right to request changes, as well as to learn who has requested access to their records.

Under Standard #2, disclosures of **protected health information (PHI)** is limited to the minimum needed for health care treatment and business operations. Patients are now able to decide if they will authorize disclosure of their **PHI** for other uses.

All **covered entities** must have a privacy policy and must notify all patients of this policy. Covered entities include hospitals; nursing homes; hospices; pharmacies; physician, dental, chiropractic, and osteopathic practices; physical therapists; alternative medicine providers; laboratories and other diagnostic centers; health care insurance plans; and health plan clearinghouses.

In addition, every covered entity must have a comprehensive compliance program in place. This written program must include a review of all health information practices to determine if there are gaps between the health information practice and the HIPAA requirements. Policies must be in place that enforce privacy. A review of all activities of the practice's business partners must be done to determine if a business associate agreement is required.

Under HIPAA, all covered entities must assign a privacy officer. This person will administer the privacy program and enforce compliance. All employees must be trained on HIPAA and the organization's privacy policies. The privacy and/or security officer must be certain that all systems provide adequate protection of patient data.

Any individual may file a complaint with the **Department of Health and Human Services Office for Civil Rights.** Figure 7.2 contains the information from the DHHS OCR about how to file a complaint.

## HOW TO FILE A HEALTH INFORMATION PRIVACY COMPLAINT WITH THE OFFICE FOR CIVIL RIGHTS

If you believe that a person agency or organization covered under the HIPAA Privacy Rule ("a covered entity") violated your (or someone else's) health information privacy rights or committed another violation of the Privacy Rule. you may file a complaint with the Office for Civil Rights (OCR). OCR has authority to receive and investigate complaints against covered entities related to the Privacy Rule. A covered entity is a health plan, health care clearinghouse, and any health care provider who conducts certain health care transactions electronically. For more information about the Privacy rule, please look at our responses to Frequently Asked Questions (FAQs) and our Privacy Guidance. (See the web link near the bottom of this form.)

Complaints to the office for Civil Rights must: (1) Be filled in writing, either on paper or electronically: (2) name the entity that is the subject of the complaint and describe the acts or omissions believed to be in violation of the applicable requirements of the Privacy Rule: and (3) be filed within 180 days of when you knew that the act of omission complained of occurred, OCR may extend the 180-day period if you can show "good cause." Any alleged violation must have occurred on or after April 14, 2003 (on or after April 14, 2004 for small health plans). for OCR to have authority to investigate.

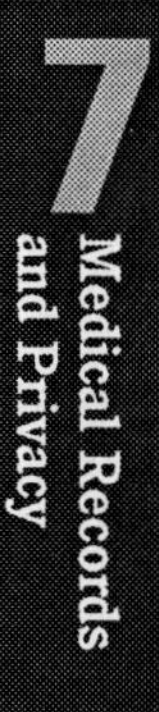


Anyone can file written complaints with OCR by mail, fax, or email. If you need help filing a complaint or have a question about the complaint form. please call this OCR toll free number: 1-800-368-1019. OCR has ten regional offices, and each regional office covers certain states. You should send your complaint to the appropriate OCR Regional Office. based on the region where the alleged violation took place. Use the OCR Regions list at the end of this Fact sheet. or you can look at the regional office map to help you determine where to send your complaint. Complaints should be sent to the attention off the appropriate OCR Regional Manager.

You can submit your complaint in any written format. We recommend that you use the OCR Health Information Privacy Complaint Form which can be found on our web site or at an OCR Regional office. If you prefer, you may submit a written complaint in your own format. Be sure to include the following information in your *written* complaint:

Your name, full address, home and work telephone numbers, email address.

If you are filling a complaint on someone's behalf, also provide the name of the person on whose behalf you are filling.

Name, full address and phone of the person, agency or organization you believe violated your (or someone else's) health Information privacy rights or committed another violation of the Privacy Rate

Briefly describe what happened. How, why and when do believe your (or someone else's) health information privacy rights were violated, or the Privacy Rule otherwise was violated?

**Figure 7.2** How to File a HIPAA Complaint (continued)

Source: Fact Sheet from the DHHS OCR, http://www.hhs.gov/ocr/hippahowtofile.pdf.

**Any other relevant information.**

**Please sign your name and date your letter.**

*The following information is optional:*

**Do you need special accommodations for us to communicate with you about this complaint?**

**If we cannot reach you directly, is there someone else we can contact to help us reach you?**

**Have you filed your complaint somewhere else?**

The Privacy Rule, developed under authority of the Health Insurance Portability and Accountability Act of 1996 (HIPAA), prohibits the alleged violating party from taking retaliatory action against anyone for filing a complaint with the Office for Civil Rights. You Should notify OCR immediately in the event of any retaliatory action. *To submit a complaint with OCR, please use one of the following methods.* If you mail or fax the complaint, be sure to follow the instructions above for determining the correct regional office.

*Option 1*: Open and print out the Health Information Privacy Complaint Form in PDF format (you will need Adobe Reader software) and fill it out. Return the completed complaint to the appropriate OCR Regional Office by mail or fax

*Option 2*: Download the Health Information Privacy Complaint Form in Microsoft Word format to your own computer, fill out and save the form using Microsoft Word. Use the Tab and Shift/Tab on your keyboard to move from field to field in the form. Then, you can either: (a) Print the completed form and mail or fax it to the appropriate OCR Regional Office; or (b) email the form to OCR at OCRComplaint@hhs.gov.

*Option 3*: If you choose not to use the OCR-provided Health Information Privacy Complaint Form (although we recommend that you do), please provide the information specified above and either (a) send a letter or fax to the appropriate OCR Regional Office: or (b) send an email OCR at OCRComplaint@hhs.gov.

If you require an answer regarding a general health information privacy question, please view our Frequently Asked Questions (FAQs). If you still need assistance, you may call OCR (toll-free) at: 1-866-627-7748. You may also send an email to OCRPrivacy@hhs.gov with suggestions regarding future FAQs. Emails will not receive individual responses.

**Figure 7.2** (concluded)



**Table 7.3** Patient Rights Under HIPAA

| Patient Right | Comments | Documentation Required | Documentation Recommended |
|---|---|---|---|
| Access to medical records and the right to copy them. | Access to records is guaranteed under HIPAA, but there are some limitations. | No. | Yes. |
| Request for amendment to designated record set. | A patient has the right to request amendments to his or her PHI or | Yes. | |

*(continued)*

**Table 7.3 Patient Rights Under HIPAA** (continued)

| Patient Right | Comments | Documentation Required | Documentation Recommended |
|---|---|---|---|
| | other personal information. Unless a provider has grounds to deny the request, amendments must be made. | | |
| Request for an accounting of disclosures of PHI. | You are required to account for certain disclosures. Check with your privacy officer for a list. You have up to 60 days to provide the disclosure list. | Yes. Always keep a record of the appropriate disclosures, and make a copy of the disclosure report for the patient's file. | |
| Request to be contacted at an alternate location. | Patients can request to have you contact them at places other than work or home. You can deny the request if you cannot reasonably comply. | Yes. Obtain a request from the patient in writing. Note in the patient's electronic medical record and in a paper communication for staff members who do not have access to the patient's electronic medical record. Document reasons for denying the request if it is denied. | |
| Requests for further restrictions on who has access to PHI. | A patient can request that certain persons or entities do not have access to his or her medical record. You may deny the request if you cannot reasonably comply. | Yes. Ask the patient to complete an opt-out form that is then filed with electronic and paper records. Document reasons for denying the request if it is denied. | |

(continued)

Table 7.3 Patient Rights Under HIPAA (concluded)

| Patient Right | Comments | Documentation Required | Documentation Recommended |
|---|---|---|---|
| Right to file a complaint. | Enforcement of the Privacy Rule is complaint-driven. Patients should be encouraged to work first with the provider. Retaliation is prohibited. | Yes. Refer the complaint to the privacy officer. Document the complaint in a privacy complaint log. Evaluate the complaint and determine how best to solve it. | |

Source: From Judson, K., Harrison, C., and Hicks, S., *Law and Ethics for Medical Careers,* 4e. Copyright © 2006 The McGraw-Hill Companies, Inc. Reprinted with permission.

HIPAA has established six important rights for patients. As an employee of a medical practice, you have a responsibility to ensure that these rights are enforced. Table 7.3 lists those rights.

The likelihood is that your practice has established all of the appropriate standards over the last several years. If for some reason it has not implemented Standard #2, there is a wealth of information available. Check the Centers for Medicare and Medicaid Services (CMS) official website for more information about HIPAA. The site's current address is http://www.cms.hhs.gov/HIPAAGenInfo/.



## Release of Information (ROI)

It is the ethical and legal responsibility of all members of the practice to maintain **confidentiality** of the patient's medical information. HIPAA may have made us think more about confidentiality, but **release of information (ROI)** has always been an ethical consideration in health care. Here are some suggestions to avoid inadvertent release of information:

- When speaking on the phone, do not use the caller's name if others in the area might overhear.
- Use caution in giving the results of medical tests to patients over the telephone to prevent others from hearing.
- Do not leave medical charts or other medical or insurance information where patients and other visitors can see them.
- Be discreet when discussing financial information with a patient. Be certain others cannot overhear your conversation.
- Be careful about discussing a patient's condition in the hallways outside exam rooms. Many times, the patients in the exam room can hear everything you are saying.

To release protected health information, it is important that you have written permission from the patient. Most practices have a standard ROI form. A sample ROI is found in Figure 7.3. Note that in the form there are special considerations for the

I authorize: Name of person or institution ____________
(Provider of information)
Street address ____________
City, state, Zip Code ____________

To release medical information to:
Name of person or institution: ____________
(Recipient of information)
Street address ____________
City, state, Zip Code ____________
Attention: ____________

Nature of information to be disclosed:
☐ Clinical notes pertaining to evaluation and treatment
☐ Other, please specify ____________

Purpose of disclosure:
☐ Continuing medical care
☐ Second opinion
☐ Other, please specify ____________

This authorization will automatically expire one year from the date of signature, unless specified otherwise ____________

This consent may be revoked at any time by sending written notice to the above-named provider of information. Any release of information made prior to the revocation of this compliant authorization is not a breach of confidentiality. Disclosed information may be reviewed by contacting the provider of information.

Patient's name ____________

Signature of patient or legal guardian ____________ Date ____________

Complete address ____________

Relationship, if not the patient ____________ Patient's date of birth ____________

SPECIFIC CONSENT FOR RELEASE OF INFORMATION
PROTECTED BY STATE OR FEDERAL LAW

Iowa law (and in some cases federal law) provides special confidentiality protection to information relating to substance abuse, mental health, and HIV-related testing. In order for information to be released on this subject matter, this specific authorization and the above authorization must be signed:

I authorize release of information relating to:

☐ Substance abuse (alcohol/drug abuse)
Signature of patient or legal guardian
____________ Date ____________

☐ Mental health (includes psychological testing and mental health counseling)
Signature of patient or legal guardian
____________ Date ____________

☐ HIV-related information (AIDS-related testing)
Signature of patient or legal guardian
____________ Date ____________

Date information is sent ____________ Sent by (name) ____________

To the recipient of this information: This information has been disclosed to you from records protected by federal confidentiality rules. The federal rules prohibit you from making further disclosure without additional consent.

Figure 7.3 Standard Release of Information (ROI) Form

release of psychotherapy notes, drug and alcohol treatment notes, and HIV/AIDS treatment notes.

## Informed Consent

**Consent** means that the patient has given permission for the physical exam, lab tests, and other medical procedures. There are three types of consent in health care: implied consent, expressed consent, and informed consent.

*Implied* consent is when by your actions you agree to be treated. When a patient makes an appointment for an examination, implied consent for the physician to perform the exam has been given. *Expressed* consent includes implied consent, but also includes the basic consent to treat forms that most patients sign.

*Informed* consent is needed for surgery and some other procedures such as a test for HIV. Implied consent is not enough in these cases. The doctrine of informed consent is the legal basis for informed consent, which is usually addressed in a state's **medical practice act.** Informed consent implies that the patient understands the following:

- Proposed modes of treatment
- Why the treatment is necessary
- Risks involved in the proposed treatment
- Available alternative modes of treatment
- Risks involved if treatment is refused



Informed consent involves the patient's right to receive all information relative to his or her condition and then make an informed decision. Informed consent also proves that the patient was not coerced into treatment. A sample informed consent form for surgery is found in Figure 7.4.

Only adults of sound mind are usually able to give informed consent. The following individuals normally cannot give informed consent:

- Minors usually cannot give informed consent. The exceptions to this include emancipated minors (those living away from home and responsible for their own support), married minors, and mature minors seeking birth control or care during pregnancy.
- Mentally incompetent patients cannot give informed consent. The patient must be judged by the court to be insane, senile, mentally disabled, or under the influence of drugs or alcohol. A competent person may be designated to give informed consent.

# INFORMED CONSENT for SURGERY and PROCEDURES

1. I hereby authorize staff physicians and resident staff at ______________________ (Name of Hospital or Facility) to perform upon ______________________ (Name of Patient), such treatment, procedures and/or operations necessary to treat or diagnose the condition(s) which appear indicated.

2. The operation(s) or procedure(s) necessary to treat and/or diagnose my condition and the risks, benefits/alternatives and options associated with them have been explained to me by ______________________ (Name of Physician or Provider), and I understand the operation(s) or procedure(s) to be: ______________________

3. **Different Provider:** ☐ Not Applicable
I understand and approve that a different provider other than the physician named above may actually perform the procedure.

4. **Operative Side:** ☐ Not Applicable ☐ Left ☐ Right

5. **Sedation & Local Anesthetics:** I authorize the administration of sedation and the use of local anesthetics, drugs and medicines as may be deemed appropriate. If they will be used, the risks and benefits/alternatives of sedation have been explained to me by the procedural physician.

6. **Blood and Blood Products:** ☐ Not Applicable
I understand certain surgeries, procedures, or illnesses may result in loss of blood. I authorize the administration of blood and/or blood components during the procedure as well as during the course of my hospital stay. If blood will be used, the risks, benefits/alternatives have been explained to me by the physician.
Patient Initials: __________

7. **No Blood Products:** ☐ Not Applicable
**I request that NO blood derivative be administered to me. I hereby release the hospital, its personnel, the attending physician and its agents from any responsibility whatsoever for unfavorable reactions or any untoward results due to my refusal to permit the use of blood or its derivatives. The possible risks and consequences of such refusal on my part have been fully explained and I fully understand such risks and consequences may occur as a result of my refusal.**
Signature of Patient/Responsible Person: ______________________ Relationship: __________

8. **Unforeseen Conditions:** It has been explained to me that during the course of the operation(s) or procedure(s) unforeseen conditions may be revealed that necessitate an extension of the original procedure(s) or different procedure(s) than those set forth above. I am aware that the practice of medicine is not an exact science and I acknowledge that no guarantees have been made to me concerning the results of this operation(s) or procedure(s).

9. **Photography:** I consent to the use of photography, closed circuit television recording and to use the photographs and other materials for study, educational and scientific purposes, in accordance with ordinary practices of the facility.

10. I consent to have my procedure/operation observed, for educational purposes, by individual(s) other than those assisting the physician during the procedure/operation.

| Physician or Provider Signature | Patient's Signature *(If competent)* | Witness | Date | Time |
|---|---|---|---|---|

| Signature of Interpreter *(If applicable)* | Date | Time | Signature of Person Responsible/Relationship | Date | Time |
|---|---|---|---|---|---|
| Witness *(Telephone consent)* **Physician must initial faxed copy** | Date | Time | Second Physician or Provider Signature for Emergencies for Incompetent Patient and No Family | Date | Time |

**Figure 7.4** Informed Consent Form

Source: From Judson, K., Harrison, C., and Hicks, S., *Law and Ethics for Medical Careers,* 4e. Copyright © 2006 The McGraw-Hill Companies, Inc. Reprinted with permission.

- Patients who speak a foreign language. Interpreters are necessary in order to inform patients of treatments.

Patient education is vital in the issue of informed consent. Just handing a patient a brochure or informed consent form to sign is not enough. Patients must be educated about the procedure they are scheduled to have. Patients who sue successfully claim lack of informed consent because they did not read the consent form they signed or did not read the patient material provided to them. Be sure your informed consent process is a thorough one.

## Summary

The medical record is the most important record that a medical practice maintains. Having at hand the appropriate documentation in a timely manner is crucial for effective patient care. A lack of information or information that is hard to find could impact the patient's care. In today's electronic environment, it is also difficult to secure the information properly to ensure the patient's privacy. All members of the medical practice must follow the appropriate guidelines for charting and the HIPAA regulations to ensure privacy. Care must be taken by all staff members to maintain confidentiality. Where informed consent is necessary, it is critical that the process be handled with sensitivity and thoroughness.

# Chapter 8

# Health Insurance

## Introduction

*The cost of health care continues to rise. Many Americans look to their health insurance or Medicare and Medicaid to help pay the costs of health care services. Health insurance coverage is complicated. Not all plans have the same coverage, and there are confusing terms such as* copayment *and* coinsurance *to understand. All staff members in the medical office need to have a basic understanding of U.S. health insurance.*

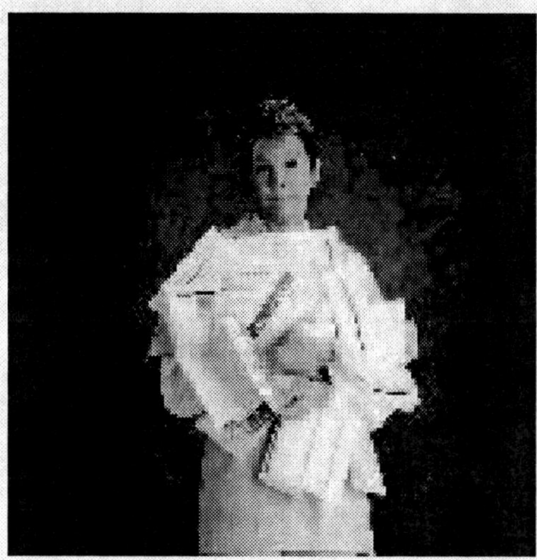

Sometimes the paperwork is overwhelming.

## Chapter Outline

## Short History of Health Insurance in the United States

The first health insurance plans in this country were established during the Civil War. These plans were not like the plans that exist today; rather, they provided coverage against accidents related to travel by train or steamboat. Some individual insurance companies began issuing disability and illness policies in the late 1800s.

The first modern group health insurance plan was formed in 1929 in Dallas. A group of teachers contracted with Baylor Hospital to cover the costs associated with having a baby delivered at the hospital. The teachers contributed fifty cents a month, and Baylor Hospital agreed to cover the cost of their room, board, and medical fees while having the baby.

In the 1930s and 1940s several large life insurance companies entered the health insurance field. In 1932 the first nonprofit organizations called Blue Cross and Blue Shield offered group health plans. These plans continued to grow, particularly as the unions bargained with employers for better benefit packages.

In 1965, Medicare and Medicaid became the first government-sponsored health insurance plans. Medicare was originally established to help cover older people, while Medicaid was for people who were very poor. The federal government had provided disability benefits through Social Security beginning in 1954.

During the 1980s and 1990s the cost of health care rose dramatically. As the actual costs increased, so did the premiums paid by employers for health insurance. In addition, the costs to Medicare and Medicaid increased rapidly. In the mid-nineties, both the federal government and employers began to look at managed care plans. A large number of people across the country were enrolled in health maintenance organizations through their employer-sponsored plans. Intended to save money, the health maintenance plans were not popular with many Americans.

Beginning in 2000, employers began to look at a variety of plans that provided more choice than health maintenance plans. Additionally, most employers began to require that employees pay a share of the cost of the premium. Most Americans that have health insurance today are enrolled in some kind of managed care plan. We will look at managed care in more detail later in the chapter.

Most experts suggest that approximately 43 million Americans in any given year are without health insurance and approximately 15% of the uninsured are children. Some of the adults are unemployed, but many are employed and unable to afford their share of the premium costs for the plans their employers offer. Efforts for universal health care in America have never been successful. Your practice's financial success is dependent on patients, their insurance companies, or Medicare or Medicaid paying the bill, so it is likely that your office limits the number of patients who do not have some kind of health insurance.

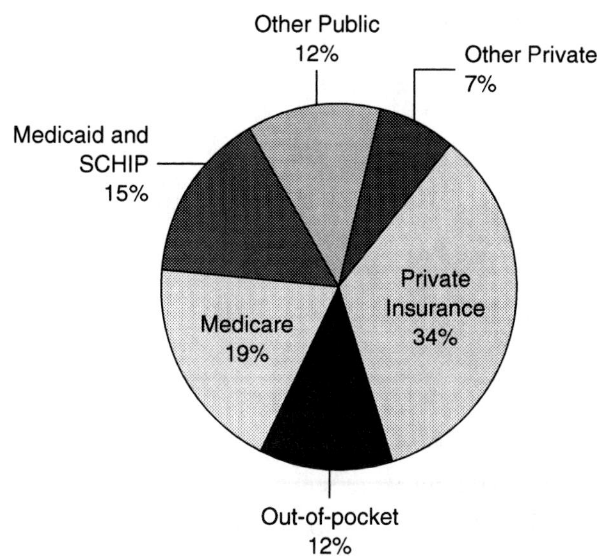


**Figure 8.1** Health Care Expenditures by Source of Funding, 2006

Source: Centers for Medicare and Medicaid Services, Office of the Actuary, National Health Statistics Group.

The cost of health care is an important issue for all Americans. The majority of health care costs are paid for by a third-party payer. Figure 8.1 reflects the source of funding for health care expenditures nationwide in 2006.

# Types of Health Insurance

Health insurance, regardless of what type it is, is a contract between the patient and the insurance company or other **third-party payer.** The contract states that the insurance company will pay a portion of your medical expenses for sicknesses and injuries. That portion of the costs to be paid by the insurance company varies with every contract. The patient (and/or the employer) agrees to pay a premium each month. There are three general types of insurance plans: group health plans, individual health policies, and government-sponsored plans. In addition, both group health plans and government-sponsored plans can be either traditional insurance or managed care. Individual coverage is almost always traditional insurance.

## Group Health Plans

A **group health plan** is any plan sponsored by an organization. Typically, group health plans are sponsored by employers, but some professional organizations offer group health plan coverage. Any person who is a member of the group is eligible to be covered by the plan. There are two types of group health plans:

- *Insured plans*—where the organization chooses either a managed care plan or traditional insurance plan.

- *Self-funded plans*—where the employer takes the risk and is itself the insurer, hiring an insurance company or other company to review claims and make payments from the employer's funds. In this case, the company paying the claims on behalf of the employer is only an agent, called a **third-party administrator.**

## Individual Health Plans

People purchase an **individual health plan** from an insurance company directly. Depending on the plan, the insurance company may require that the insured pay the claim first and be reimbursed by the insurance company, or the plan may operate like a group plan and pay the physicians and other parties directly. Individual plans are usually expensive and come with a high deductible. They may have features similar to managed care plans, or they may resemble indemnity plans.

An **indemnity plan** allows the insured to choose any provider without effect on reimbursement. However, most indemnity plans use the usual, customary and reasonable (UCR) principle in determining appropriate charges to be reimbursed. More information about UCR is found later in the chapter. Obtaining indemnity coverage for health care is difficult and expensive, as most insurance companies prefer to use at least a preferred provider network.

All patients are issued a card that provides basic information to the providers. A sample card is shown in Figure 8.2.

## Managed Care Plans

The terms *managed care* plan and *health maintenance organization* are often used interchangeably. They are different, however. **Managed care** is a general term referring to any health care plan that is not an indemnity plan (i.e., any plan that has some kind of restrictions on which providers the insured may use). Managed care plans include preferred provider

McGraw Insurance Companies — BlueMed

Tawney Johnson
Contract No. XJW651-552973

| GROUP NO. | BM PLAN |
|---|---|
| 9999PP3 | 909 |

Customer Service No. 800-555-6757
Send claims to: PO Box 55, Cityville, FL 32901

FRONT OF CARD

| Type Contract | GROUP | |
|---|---|---|
| Type Coverage | GROUP | |
| | PPO | NON_PPO |
| Co-Insurance | 80% | 60% |
| Deductible | ------$2,000----- | |
| Hospital per Adm Deductible | $0 | $500 |
| Family Physician Office Svs | $15co-pay | 60% |
| All Other Physician Svs | 80% | 60% |

Admission Certification Required Call 800-555-5971
24-month Preexisting Condition Limitation

BACK OF CARD

**Figure 8.2** Insurance Card

Source: From Safian, S., *Insurance Coding and Electronic Claims,* p. 41. Copyright © The McGraw-Hill Companies, Inc. Reprinted with permission.

organizations, exclusive provider organizations, health maintenance organizations, and point of service plans. All these type of plans manage care, but they have different restrictions in place. A health maintenance organization is a specific type of managed care.

**Preferred provider organization (PPO)** plans provide coverage through a network of selected health care providers (physicians and hospitals). The insured may go outside the network, but would pay more of the costs for care. Some PPOs have higher deductibles and higher coinsurance payments when the insured goes out of network.

**Exclusive provider organization (EPO)** plans are a more restrictive type of PPO. The insured must use providers from a specified network of physicians and hospitals to receive coverage. There is no coverage for care received from a nonnetwork provider unless it is an emergency.

A **health maintenance organization (HMO)** is a health care system that assumes both the financial risk associated with providing comprehensive medical services (the insurance) and the responsibility for health care delivery in a particular geographic area (the care). Thus, an HMO is both an insurer and a provider. The insured may not use non-HMO providers unless it is an emergency. However, even in an emergency most HMOs strongly encourage their insured to use the hospitals in the HMO network. Individuals belonging to an HMO are not responsible for their bill as long as they see HMO physicians. Most HMOs have a copayment requirement. Usually there is no deductible or coinsurance. Depending on the plan, the insured individuals may not go to a specialist within the HMO without a referral from their primary physician.

HMOs deliver services in one of two ways: They may have their own facilities and physicians, or they may contract with group practices and hospitals to provide services. In the latter type of arrangement, the physicians and hospitals may also provide services to non-HMO patients.

## Government-Sponsored Plans

Our federal and state governments sponsor a variety of health care coverage. Of course, the most well known are Medicare and Medicaid; however, workers' compensation, TRICARE, and CHAMPVA are also government sponsored.

Both Medicare and Medicaid plans have been in existence since the mid-sixties. There are major differences between the two programs. The first thing to keep in mind is that Medicare is an insurance program, whereas Medicaid is an assistance program.

**Medicare** is a federal program financed through both general income taxes and the Medicare payroll withholding tax. The current withholding tax is 1.45% of earnings. The employer must also match that contribution. Medical bills are paid from trust funds created by the withholding tax.

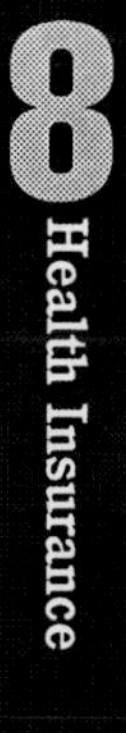

Medicare is for people over 65, whatever their income. It also serves younger people who are disabled and individuals undergoing dialysis. Patients pay part of the costs through deductibles for hospital and other costs. Monthly premiums are required for nonhospital coverage. As mentioned, Medicare is a federal program. With the exception of Medicare Part C, it is basically the same everywhere in the United States. The rules and regulations are set by the **Centers for Medicare and Medicaid Services (CMS),** an agency of the federal Department of Health and Human Services. Every enrollee is issued a card with the enrollment information on it.

Medicare has four parts. *Part A* covers hospital services and inpatient stays in a skilled nursing facility. The nursing home care must be inpatient in nature; Medicare does not cover custodial or long-term care in a nursing home. Additionally, hospice care services and some home health care services are covered. Although there are some limits to what Medicare will cover, there is no premium for Part A if you or your spouse paid Medicare taxes while working.

*Part B* Medicare covers doctors' services, outpatient care, some other medical services Part A does not cover, and some preventive services. A monthly premium must be paid. In 2008 that premium was $96.40 a month. Your premium may be higher if your income (single) is more than $82,000 annually. In addition, depending on which type of service and which type of plan chosen, you may have to pay a coinsurance and a deductible. Your costs may be different if you are a member of a Medicare Advantage Program (Part C of Medicare) or you have other insurance like a **Medigap** policy or employer coverage.

*Part C* coverage from Medicare is called the Medicare Advantage Program. This program is the managed care portion of Medicare. Recipients may elect to join a Part C provider in lieu of Part B and sometimes Part D. The plans in the Medicare Advantage Plans are run in a similar manner to other managed care plans. Recipients may receive better benefits from a Medicare Advantage Plan, depending on the plan selected.

The last part of Medicare is Medicare *Part D,* which is the prescription drug benefit. There are a variety of plans in the marketplace. Some of these plans work in conjunction with Part C.

Medicare coverage is complicated. It is important for the patient to access the government's website, medicare.gov, for the latest information. Practices should access the Centers for Medicare and Medicaid Services website (www.cms.hhs.gov/) for updated provider information. Staying informed is the best practice.

**Medicaid** is an assistance program, not an insurance plan. Individuals must be eligible for assistance, based on income and other criteria. They may be eligible one month and not eligible the next month. Medical bills are paid from federal, state, and local tax funds. Medicaid serves a select group of low-income people. Patients usually pay no part of the costs for covered medical expenses. A small copayment is sometimes required, but no premium payment is required. Medicaid is a federal-state program and varies from state to state. It is run by state and local governments within federal guidelines. Medicaid rules and payments differ from state to state, so if your practice accepts Medicaid, a member of the billing staff should monitor the state's Medicaid website for changes and updates. Many providers are reluctant to accept Medicaid patients because the reimbursement rate is so low. Additionally, Medicaid limits what it will pay for.

The **State Children's Health Insurance (SCHIP)** covers uninsured children under the age of 19 whose families earn a certain amount ($36,200 for a family of four in 2007). For little or no cost, SCHIP pays for doctor visits, hospitalizations, immunizations, and emergency room visits. Families who earn too much to qualify for Medicaid may be able to qualify for SCHIP.

There are two other forms of health insurance provided by either the federal or individual state governments. One is specifically for the military and their families, while the other covers workers injured on the job.

In 1966, Congress created the Civilian Health and Medical Program of the Uniformed Services (CHAMPUS). This federally funded program provided comprehensive health benefits for dependents of active-duty military personnel and dependents of military personnel who died while on active duty as well as retired military personnel and their dependents. In 1993, CHAMPUS became **TRICARE.** The TRICARE system has three choices for military families. These choices are:

- *TRICARE Standard*—this is similar to an indemnity plan and is often referred to as the old CHAMPUS plan. Patients have more choice in providers, but they pay a higher out-of-pocket cost.
- *TRICARE Extra*—this is similar to a PPO in that patients must obtain their care from an approved list of providers.
- *TRICARE Prime*—this plan is similar to an HMO in that patients are assigned a primary case manager and all care is coordinated through the case manager. It is the least expensive of the options.

There are several other types of plans under the TRICARE umbrella that provide care for beneficiaries who are Medicare eligible or who receive care only at military facilities.

TRICARE divides the country into three regions for administration of the TRICARE plan. Providers should access http://tricare.mil, and click on the Providers button to obtain up-to-date information on rules and regulations for participation and filing of claims for their region.


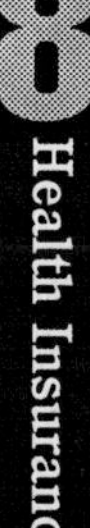

TRICARE is for active-duty and retired members of the uniformed services, their families, and survivors. It is different from the **Civilian Health and Medical Program of the Department of Veterans Affairs (CHAMPVA).** As indicated by its name, CHAMPVA is administered by the Department of Veterans Affairs. TRICARE and CHAMPVA are often mistaken for one another, but they are separately administered by different parts of the federal government. According to the Department of Veterans Affairs, you cannot participate as a member in both TRICARE and CHAMPVA.

To be eligible for CHAMPVA, you cannot be eligible for TRICARE and you must be in one of these categories:

- The spouse or child of a veteran who has been rated permanently and totally disabled for a service-connected disability by a VA regional office.
- The surviving spouse or child of a veteran who died from a VA-rated service-connected disability.
- The surviving spouse or child of a veteran who at the time of death was rated permanently and totally disabled from a service-connected disability.
- The surviving spouse or child of a military member who died in the line of duty, not due to misconduct. Most of the time, these survivors are eligible for TRICARE, not CHAMPUS.

Under TRICARE and CHAMPVA, the insured is called the **beneficiary.** Also, TRICARE and CHAMPVA are considered secondary benefits when the patient is eligible for Medicare.

**Workers' compensation** covers health care costs for an injury or illness related to a person's job. Employers in each state pay a premium into a state fund. The premium is based on the number of employees and previous workers' compensation claims. In most states, employees are limited as to which physicians, hospitals, and other services they may use. Employees normally do not pay a premium for workers' compensation insurance.

Whenever a patient comes in with an injury, it is important to find out if the patient was injured on the job. Although most states use managed care principles to administer workers' compensation, not all workers may understand that they must report the injury or illness to their employer. Each state administers workers' compensation differently. For providers, it is important to know the state's rules. Some basics for workers' compensation claims are outlined in Table 8.1.

The many types of third-party payment make it necessary for everyone to stay current on the various rules and regulations. Although it is not a separate type of insurance, there is one more term that is important in considering sources or types of insurance.

The **Consolidated Omnibus Budget Reconciliation Act (COBRA)** of 1985 was set up to allow individuals to continue their employer-sponsored health insurance for a limited

Table 8.1 Workers' Compensation Documentation Management

- A first report of injury must be filed with the employer, the employer's identified workers' compensation insurance carrier, and the state workers' compensation board, as well as the patient's medical record.
- Care must be taken not to release any other information in the patient's file that is unrelated to the workers' compensation claim. The employer and the state are entitled to information about treatment for the work-related injury or illness only.
- A progress report (or reports) must be filed on a routine basis. Each state may have specific requirements, but at a minimum, the treatment and progress, a statement regarding continued need for treatment, estimate of patient status regarding return to work, and any outside reports (lab, X-ray, or consultants) should be included in the report.
- A final report should be prepared as appropriate providing the final medical status regarding permanent disability, expressed as percentage of loss of function.
- THE CMS-1500 form (discussed in detail in Chapter 10) should always reflect that the care provided is a workers' compensation matter.

amount of time after losing a job. Individuals may have COBRA coverage for 18 months and possibly up to 36 months, depending on the circumstances of the employment termination and any disability. The employee must pay the premium. Since the coverage is identical to what patients had before they became unemployed, the change may be transparent to the practice. As is discussed in Chapter 10, timely claims filing is important because that may be the first time the practice learns the patient no longer has coverage. Many practices have the ability to check online to verify active coverage. Done before the patient is seen may help avoid an embarrassing moment for all concerned.

## Types of Health Insurance Payments

Like everything else in the health care business, payment is not necessarily a straightforward event. Understanding the various payment mechanisms involved is important, particularly when a patient asks about it. Some of the payment process is covered in Chapter 10, but let's look at a few payment basics.

### Fee-for-Service

Indemnity plans are essentially **fee-for-service** plans. The insurance company reimburses the provider or patient for all or part of the services. Covered services are those services that by contract the insurance company has agreed to pay. However, the insurance company has not necessarily agreed to pay the charges the provider submits.

There is a concept in the health insurance reimbursement arena called **usual, customary and reasonable (UCR)** charges. This means that in fee-for-service coverage, an insurance company may determine that the charges of a physician are above UCR. When this happens, the insurance company will pay only its share of what it determines to be usual, customary and reasonable. For example, a provider may charge $100 for a particular service. If the patient has an 80–20 plan, the patient pays $20 and the insurance company pays $80, assuming that the deductible has been met. However, the insurance company may have determined that $75 is the UCR charge for that service. If that is the case, the insurance company will pay 80% of the $75, or $60, and the patient is responsible for the balance of $40.

## Preferred Provider Organization Payments

If the provider is a participating preferred provider organization (PPO), the normal charge is billed but the provider has agreed to accept a lower payment and bill the patient only for the balance due on the lower amount. Using the previous example, if the physician is a participating provider, then the patient would pay $15. This is the coinsurance, not the copayment. The terms *copayment* and *coinsurance* are often confusing.

In PPO plans, there is also a sharing of the costs of covered care between the patient and the insurance company. The plan might be an 80–20 plan. That means that the insurance company will cover 80% of the covered charges, with the patient responsible for the 20% of charges. This percentage amount is called **coinsurance.** The difference between the fee-for-service and preferred provider reimbursement is that there has been a negotiated agreement between the insurance company and the provider as to the accepted payment. The patient is responsible for the coinsurance of the negotiated amount, not the actual charge.

**Copayments** are a flat fee that the patient is expected to pay for each visit or service. Copayments differ depending on the service. As an example, the copay for an office visit and a prescription may be different. Some services may have no copay. Copayments are not a part of the coinsurance.

Medicare, Medicaid, workers' compensation, and the various military plans usually function as PPOs when it comes to payment. However, there are exceptions. The business office of your medical practice should be familiar with those exceptions.

## Deductibles

Most insurance plans, whether indemnity, PPO, or Medicare, have a deductible. A **deductible** is the out-of-pocket costs the patient is expected to pay before the health insurance begins. Most deductibles are on an annual basis and most, but not all, are on a calendar year. The amount of the deductible is specified in the insurance plan. There are some services that may be exempt from the deductible. For example, some insurance plans cover an annual physical regardless of whether the deductible has been met. The deductible can be as low as $250 or as high as $5,000, depending on the plan. Most individual plans have high deductibles in an attempt to keep down the premium cost.

## Health Maintenance Organization Payments

HMOs are not like the other forms of insurance. Remember that the HMO is not only the provider of care, but the insurer also. Your practice may or may not be part of an HMO, and there are a variety of ways your practice may be participating in an HMO. Table 8.2 lists the various models of HMO participation.

If your practice does participate in an HMO, there are several ways the practice may be paid. **Capitation** is the first method. In capitation, the providers are reimbursed a predetermined fixed amount per member per month (PMPM). The practice has been assigned a certain number of members for care. The practice is paid the same amount PMPM, whether the member is seen in the practice once a month, 10 times a month, or not at all. The member may also have to pay a copayment for each visit, depending on the plan. Usually, only large multispecialty practices participate in this type of payment plan, but some large single-specialty plans may also participate.

The second type of payment from HMOs is a model similar to the preferred provider payment. In this case, the practice is reimbursed by the HMO for actual services provided

**Table 8.2** Health Maintenance Organization Structures

- Group Model HMO—the HMO contracts with a single-multispecialty medical group to provide care to the HMOs membership. The group may work exclusively for the HMO, or continue to see patients outside the HMO membership. The group is paid on a capitation basis.
- Staff Model HMO—this is a closed panel HMO. The physicians and other providers are employees of the HMO. Only HMO patients are seen by the physicians.
- Network Model HMO—the HMO contracts with multiple physician groups to provide services to HMO members. It may involve both single and multispecialty groups. The physicians may provide services to non-HMO members.
- Individual Practice Association (IPA) HMO—independent physicians band together to contract their services to an HMO. The physicians are not necessarily members of a group practice. Physicians may see non-HMO patients.

at a negotiated rate that is usually much less than the standard charges for the services. Again, there may be a member copayment for each visit.

The biggest difference is that the patient or member does not receive a bill. That does not mean that the visits are unaccounted for in the practice's financial system, only that the patient does not receive a bill for services, unless he or she did not make a copayment at time of service. The other instances where the patient may receive a bill is when the service is not covered, or if the member is no longer enrolled in the HMO plan.

### Cash Payments

Cash is the last type of payment. If the provider does not accept a specific insurance, the patient should pay the charges directly to the physician at the time of service. The patient completes an insurance claim form and sends the form to the insurance company for reimbursement. If the provider accepts a specific insurance, then it is the provider's responsibility to file the claim form to collect the portion of the charge that the insurance company is paying and charge the patient for the remainder. Usually, providers have an office policy that states that patients must pay their share at the time of service. Additionally, patients should always pay their copayment at time of service.

## Explanation of Benefits

As evident by the previous discussion, getting paid for services rendered in a medical office is not always an easy process. How does the provider know if the amount paid is correct? How does the billing staff know the correct amount to bill the patient, if anything? How does the patient know what was paid and is owed?

All third-party payers generate an **explanation of benefits (EOB)** that explains how the reimbursement was determined, or why the reimbursement was denied. An EOB is always sent to the patient and to the provider. The provider's EOB is a summary of all benefits paid to the provider for all claims filed during a certain period of time. It is usually called a **remittance voucher** or **remittance advice.** A sample remittance voucher is shown in Figure 8.3. As you can see, a variety of patients are listed on the remittance voucher.

The patient also receives an EOB. The EOB for the patient summarizes how the insurance company determined the reimbursement for the services received. Figure 8.4 is a sample EOB for a patient. EOBs for patients are clearly marked with the statement "This Is Not a Bill."

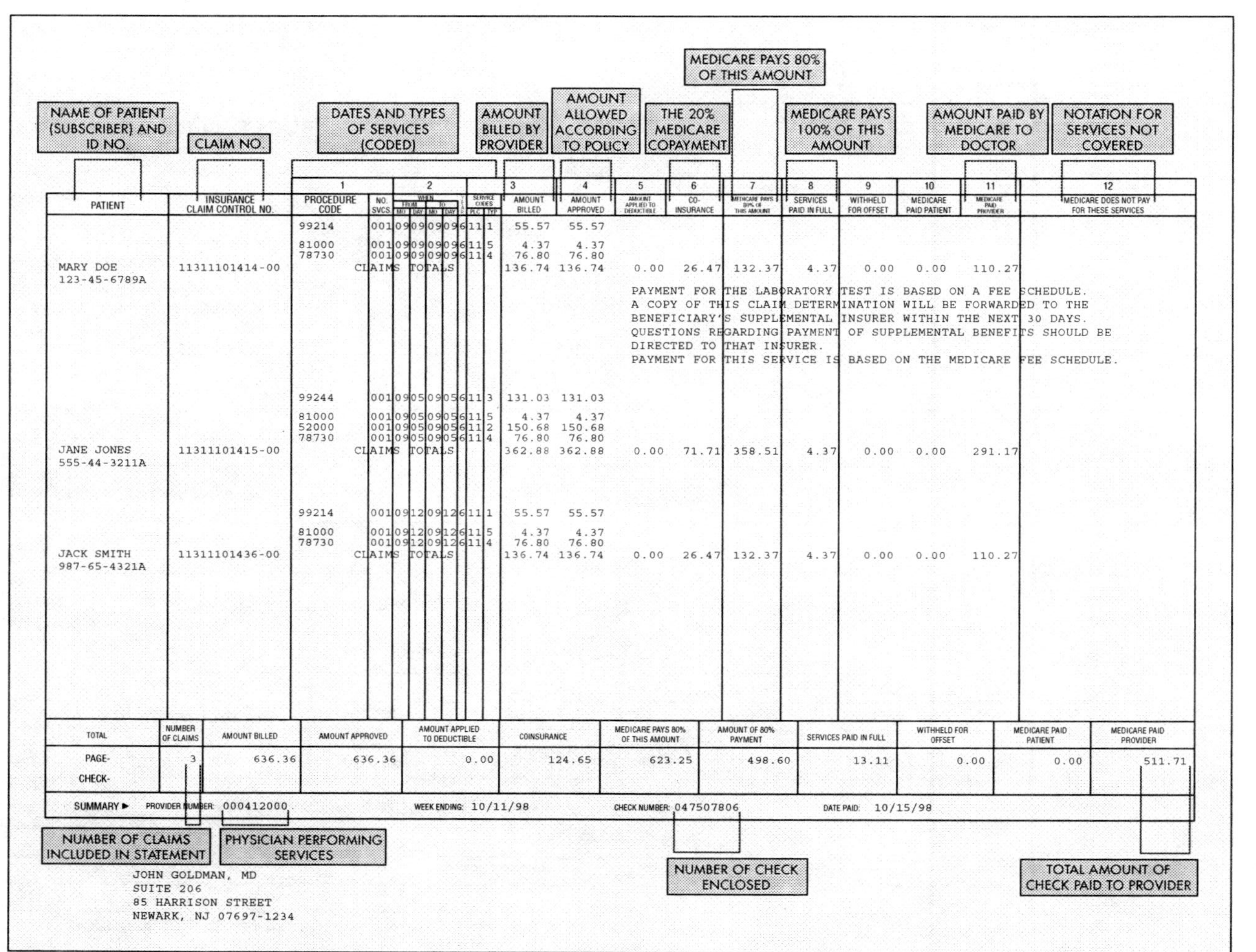


| PATIENT | INSURANCE CLAIM CONTROL NO. | 1 PROCEDURE CODE | NO. SVCS | 2 WHEN FROM MO | DAY | TO MO | DAY | YEAR | SERVICE CODES PLC | TYP | 3 AMOUNT BILLED | 4 AMOUNT APPROVED | 5 AMOUNT APPLIED TO DEDUCTIBLE | 6 CO-INSURANCE | 7 MEDICARE PAYS 80% OF THIS AMOUNT | 8 SERVICES PAID IN FULL | 9 WITHHELD FOR OFFSET | 10 MEDICARE PAID PATIENT | 11 MEDICARE PAID PROVIDER | 12 MEDICARE DOES NOT PAY FOR THESE SERVICES |
|---|---|---|---|---|---|---|---|---|---|---|---|---|---|---|---|---|---|---|---|---|
| | | 99214 | 001 | 09 | 09 | 09 | 09 | 6 | 11 | 1 | 55.57 | 55.57 | | | | | | | | |
| | | 81000 | 001 | 09 | 09 | 09 | 09 | 6 | 11 | 5 | 4.37 | 4.37 | | | | | | | | |
| | | 78730 | 001 | 09 | 09 | 09 | 09 | 6 | 11 | 4 | 76.80 | 76.80 | | | | | | | | |
| MARY DOE 123-45-6789A | 11311101414-00 | CLAIMS TOTALS | | | | | | | | | 136.74 | 136.74 | 0.00 | 26.47 | 132.37 | 4.37 | 0.00 | 0.00 | 110.27 | |
| | | 99244 | 001 | 09 | 05 | 09 | 05 | 6 | 11 | 3 | 131.03 | 131.03 | | | | | | | | |
| | | 81000 | 001 | 09 | 05 | 09 | 05 | 6 | 11 | 5 | 4.37 | 4.37 | | | | | | | | |
| | | 52000 | 001 | 09 | 05 | 09 | 05 | 6 | 11 | 2 | 150.68 | 150.68 | | | | | | | | |
| | | 78730 | 001 | 09 | 05 | 09 | 05 | 6 | 11 | 4 | 76.80 | 76.80 | | | | | | | | |
| JANE JONES 555-44-3211A | 11311101415-00 | CLAIMS TOTALS | | | | | | | | | 362.88 | 362.88 | 0.00 | 71.71 | 358.51 | 4.37 | 0.00 | 0.00 | 291.17 | |
| | | 99214 | 001 | 09 | 12 | 09 | 12 | 6 | 11 | 1 | 55.57 | 55.57 | | | | | | | | |
| | | 81000 | 001 | 09 | 12 | 09 | 12 | 6 | 11 | 5 | 4.37 | 4.37 | | | | | | | | |
| | | 78730 | 001 | 09 | 12 | 09 | 12 | 6 | 11 | 4 | 76.80 | 76.80 | | | | | | | | |
| JACK SMITH 987-65-4321A | 11311101436-00 | CLAIMS TOTALS | | | | | | | | | 136.74 | 136.74 | 0.00 | 26.47 | 132.37 | 4.37 | 0.00 | 0.00 | 110.27 | |

PAYMENT FOR THE LABORATORY TEST IS BASED ON A FEE SCHEDULE.
A COPY OF THIS CLAIM DETERMINATION WILL BE FORWARDED TO THE BENEFICIARY'S SUPPLEMENTAL INSURER WITHIN THE NEXT 30 DAYS.
QUESTIONS REGARDING PAYMENT OF SUPPLEMENTAL BENEFITS SHOULD BE DIRECTED TO THAT INSURER.
PAYMENT FOR THIS SERVICE IS BASED ON THE MEDICARE FEE SCHEDULE.

| TOTAL | NUMBER OF CLAIMS | AMOUNT BILLED | AMOUNT APPROVED | AMOUNT APPLIED TO DEDUCTIBLE | COINSURANCE | MEDICARE PAYS 80% OF THIS AMOUNT | AMOUNT OF 80% PAYMENT | SERVICES PAID IN FULL | WITHHELD FOR OFFSET | MEDICARE PAID PATIENT | MEDICARE PAID PROVIDER |
|---|---|---|---|---|---|---|---|---|---|---|---|
| PAGE- CHECK- | 3 | 636.36 | 636.36 | 0.00 | 124.65 | 623.25 | 498.60 | 13.11 | 0.00 | 0.00 | 511.71 |

SUMMARY ▸ PROVIDER NUMBER: 000412000 WEEK ENDING: 10/11/98 CHECK NUMBER: 047507806 DATE PAID: 10/15/98

JOHN GOLDMAN, MD
SUITE 206
85 HARRISON STREET
NEWARK, NJ 07697-1234

**Figure 8.3** Remittance Voucher (Explanation of Benefits for Providers)

Source: From Booth et al., *Medical Assisting,* 3e, p. 303. Copyright © 2005 The McGraw-Hill Companies, Inc. Reprinted with permission.

**BENEFITS SUMMARY - MORE HOUSE INSURANCE**

| **Patient: CARLENE HARRISON** | |
|---|---|
| **Member Number:** | **Claim Number:** |

Charges

**Itemized Charges and Paid Amounts**

| From Date of Service | To Date of Service | Description of service | Amount Billed | Allowed Amount | Deductible Amount | Copayment Amount | Coinsurance Amount | Amount Paid | You Owe | Remarks |
|---|---|---|---|---|---|---|---|---|---|---|
| 05/14/2008 | 05/14/2008 | OFFICE OR OTHER | $76.00 | $67.76 | $0.00 | $60.00 | $0.00 | $7.76 | $60.00 | 1,2 |
| | | TOTAL | $76.00 | $67.76 | $0.00 | $60.00 | $0.00 | $7.76 | $60.00 | |

Not Paid

**Amounts shown below not paid under the terms of your Benefit Booklet**

| Remarks | Explanation | Amount |
|---|---|---|
| 1 | Copayment Required for In-Network Provider | $60.00 |
| 2 | In network provider utilized. Therefore no patient responsibility. | $8.24 |
| | **TOTAL** | $68.24 |

**Accumulator Summary**
CARLENE has satisfied $0.00 of the $0.00 Deductible
HARRISON family has satisfied $0.00 of the $0.00 family Deductible
CARLENE has satisfied $60.00 of the $3,000.00 family Out of Pocket
HARRISON family has satisfied $60.00 of the $6,000.00 family Out of Pocket

Payment may include interest for claims that were not paid timely.

**Figure 8.4** Explanation of Benefits for Patients

## Other Important Insurance Terms

The language of health insurance is always challenging. There are a several other important terms that you should be familiar with when talking about insurance.

**Assignment of benefits.** This is the term used to identify who will actually receive the payment for services rendered. Patients routinely "assign" their benefits from their health insurance plan to their physician. In some cases, physicians will not see patients who do not assign their benefits.

**Balance billing.** After the insurance payment has been applied and any required adjustments are made, the patient is billed for the balance owed. Depending on the insurance plan, there may be a zero balance.

**Birthday rule.** In the past when health insurance was more affordable, both parents often covered their children through their individual insurance plans from their place of employment. In effect, the children had double coverage. To determine which plan was primary and to avoid paying claims at greater than 100%, the insurance industry developed the birthday rule. Usually, the birthday rule says that the parent with the earlier birth date (not year) was the primary for purposes of payment. In other words, if Mom's birth date is April 2 and Dad's birth date is May 3, Mom's policy is the primary policy. The rule is also used in coordination of benefits when necessary.

**Clean claim.** A clean claim is an insurance claim filed without any errors. Something as simple as reversing two numbers within a policy number can result in the claim being rejected. Clean claims are paid more quickly.

**Coordination of benefits (COB).** When a patient has more than one health insurance plan that covers services rendered, the payments are coordinated so that the total amount of the bill is not exceeded. For example, if an employee is over 65 and enrolled in Medicare as well as his or her company's health insurance, Medicare is the primary coverage. After Medicare has paid its share, the employee's health plan usually pays the balance of the approved charges.

**Gatekeeper.** In the managed care environment, a primary care physician is often designated as the gatekeeper for the patient's care. The role of the gatekeeper is to approve and make referrals to other physicians. This concept has not worked well other than in HMOs.

**Medigap.** A supplemental insurance plan for Medicare recipients that provides coverage for services, deductibles, and coinsurance not covered by Medicare. Medigap coverage is obtained from private insurance companies, not through Medicare. However, Medicare has established standards for policies that are marketed as Medigap.

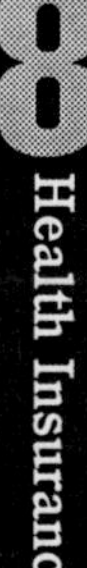

**National provider identifier (NPI).** All physicians and other providers have numerical identification numbers used to submit claims. NPI is a unique number assigned to each physician by CMS and is expected to be in full use by May 2008. Other insurance carriers are expected to begin using NPI also. Eventually, NPI is supposed to eliminate using either an employer identification number (EIN), Social Security number, or the old provider identification number (PIN). The use of one number to identify the provider to all third-party payers is the ultimate goal.

**Nonparticipating provider (nonPAR).** A physician who does not contract with Medicare and other insurance plans to accept agreed-upon amounts for services rendered. Patients are expected to pay at time of service, or to work out payment arrangements with the practice.

**Participating provider (PAR).** A PAR is a physician who contracts with Medicare and other insurance plans and agrees to accept a certain amount for services rendered. When participating with Medicare, the CMS sets the reimbursement rates at the beginning of each year. There is no negotiation. With private insurance companies, there may be some negotiation, but the insurance companies have the advantage in any negotiations.

**Preauthorization, precertification, and predetermination.** These terms always create confusion. Table 8.3 illustrates the differences. The terms defined in Table 8.3 are all similar, but they are specific and different in their application for eligibility for services.

**Preexisting conditions.** A preexisting condition is a medical condition the patient had before insurance coverage began. Depending on the plan, the patient, and the

**Table 8.3** Preauthorization, Precertification, and Predetermination

- Preauthorization—determines the medical necessity of the treatment and whether services are covered.
- Precertification—determines if a treatment is covered by a specific insurance plan for payment.
- Predetermination—defines the maximum amount of money the carrier will pay for a specific service. This is usually done in surgical cases to include surgery, consultations, and postoperative care.

condition, services provided to treat that preexisting condition may or may not be covered by the insurance plan.

**Premium.** The premium is the amount paid on a monthly, quarterly, or annual basis for health insurance. In the workplace, the cost of the premium is usually shared by the employer and employee.

**Primary and secondary coverage.** Primary coverage is the first payer when more than one insurance plan is involved. Usually the primary payer establishes the appropriate fee to be reimbursed and pays the majority percentage. The secondary payer usually is responsible for the balance. The other way that primary and secondary coverage is applied is when there is limited coverage from the primary insurance plan. For example, many auto insurance plans have limited coverage for medical costs associated with the accident. Once all of those benefits are exhausted, the patient's health insurance becomes primary. However, depending on who is at fault, coverage can become very complicated.

**Waiver or rider.** This term refers to an addendum to a health insurance policy that excludes certain conditions from coverage.

## Summary

Unlike other types of insurance, health insurance is fairly complicated. Also, unlike other types of insurance, people often don't have choices about which health insurance to purchase. Working through the complicated payment methods is often frustrating to patients. Every member of the practice should take responsibility to understand the basics of insurance so that they are able to answer patient questions. Those basics include the following:

- Knowing the difference between charges and payments.
- Understanding the basics of how health insurance plans work (not the details of each company).
- Understanding the basics of Medicare and Medicaid.
- Knowing the difference between copayments and coinsurance.
- If the practice accepts workers' compensation, understanding how it works is important.

It is unlikely that the United States will provide universal health care in the near future. Consequently, every staff member needs to have a fundamental understanding of how health insurance works.Sometimes the paperwork is overwhelming.

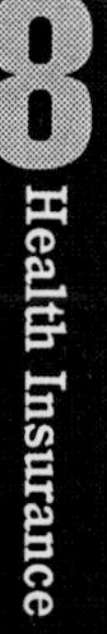

Chapter 9

# Essentials of Coding

## Introduction

*The business of health care sometimes seems like a big bowl of alphabet soup. You will hear the terms* CPT *code,* ICD-9 *code, and* HCPCS *(hic-picks) used by the business office staff, physicians, and support staff. They may be complaining that a claim was not paid because it had the wrong code. Since getting paid for the services rendered in your office is critical, it is important that everyone has a basic understanding of the various codes used to bill third-party payers for the services rendered.*

## Chapter Outline

## The Purpose of Coding

Why do we use codes? First, the federal government mandates that all providers use the same codes to bill for the same services. The Health Insurance Portability and Accountability Act (HIPAA) required a national standard code set for procedures. This is not only to ensure consistency, but to hopefully help eliminate fraud. Accurate coding helps in getting proper payment for health care provided. Incorrect or inaccurate coding can lead to investigations of fraud and abuse.

Second, coding is a way to collect data about the state of the country's health care. If we read a report or hear in a news program that there were 234,000 hip replacement surgeries done in the United States in 2004, how does the author of that report know that number? You can check for that kind of information with the **National Center for Health Statistics (NCHS),** an agency within the **Centers for Disease Control and Prevention (CDC).** That type of information is routinely provided by third-party payers to the NCHS so that, as a country, we have a sense of the health of the nation. The payers don't report who had the hip replacement surgery, only how many were done. If the payers had to report all of that information, it would be difficult to collect the data.

A third reason for using codes is that they make it easier to submit claims for service. Additionally, accurate coding provides researchers with information for epidemiological studies and quality of care issues.

There are really two types of coding that are commonly used to describe what was done for the patient and why. Understanding the types of coding is important for all staff members of the medical office. Although the providers and the billing staff must have a more detailed understanding of the coding system, all staff need to know the basics.

The **Healthcare Common Procedure Coding System (HCPCS)** was developed by the **Centers for Medicare and Medicaid Services (CMS)** for use when coding services provided to Medicare patients. Level I HCPCS codes consist of the CPT codes. Level II codes are called national codes, and they cover such things as supplies, drugs, and **durable medical equipment (DME).** It is important to remember that HCPCS codes are now in use with all insurance providers, not just Medicare and Medicaid.

As stated, **Current Procedural Terminology (CPT)** codes are Level I HCPCS codes. CPT codes tell the payers what procedures were done by the physician or other health care provider. The service may consist of a simple office visit, or it may be major surgery. It could be a lab test or a complicated invasive test. Whatever the procedure, there is a code for it.

Level II HCPCS codes are commonly referred to as HCPCS codes. These codes are used to identify materials used or given to the patient. HCPCS codes are also codes for services

*Note:* Information in this chapter was taken from *Current Procedural Terminology (CPT) 2007,* American Medical Association. 

like dental care. Many of the codes are used only by specific contractors with Medicare or Medicaid. Level II HCPCS are alphanumerical listing of codes that are not covered in Level I CPT. Some of the most commonly used HCPCS codes in the medical office are for injections and supplies.

The **International Classification of Diseases, Ninth Revision (ICD-9)** tells "why" the health care provider did the procedure and is the second type of coding. This is the diagnosis code. Often patients have more than one diagnosis. All diagnoses related to the visit or session must be provided to the payer. The ICD-9 and the CPT must be linked. For example, if the patient had a mammogram (CPT code 76092), then the diagnosis should be related to the procedure. The patient's diagnosis should be one that reflects the reason for the mammogram. If there was a mass or lump in the breast, 611.72 would be the appropriate code. But, if it was a screening mammogram, the appropriate ICD-9 code would be V76.12.

Let's look at the individual coding systems and how to use them.

## Current Procedural Terminology (CPT)

As stated previously, CPT codes describe the procedures and services performed by physicians and other health care providers. The *Current Procedural Terminology,* Fourth Edition (CPT) is revised by the American Medical Association annually. Your office should always have at least one copy of the most recent edition on hand. Usually you will find them in the practice's business office, as well as at the check-out desk. Often, a third copy is kept near the medical assistants' or nurses' station in the exam room area. The new code books are usually available in October of each year for the following year.

Each service or procedure is identified with a five-digit code. This simple coding makes the reporting of services easier for everyone.

The *Current Procedural Terminology,* Fourth Edition (CPT) is divided into six sections. Each of those sections is divided into subsections with anatomic, procedural, condition, or descriptor headings. The procedures and services are listed in numeric order, but there is one big exception to the numeric order.

Evaluation and Management (E&M) codes (99201–99499) are listed first in the *Current Procedural Terminology,* Fourth Edition (CPT). The reason is that these codes are used most often by physicians and other health care providers. Evaluation of the patient's problem and his or her medical management is the most frequent type of procedure done by physicians and other providers.

The E&M section is divided into categories such as office visit, hospital visit, and consultation. Most codes distinguish between new and established patients, except for emergency room visits. Selecting the appropriate level of evaluation and management procedures is very important. The introductory pages of the E&M section have specific instructions. Although it is the provider's responsibility to decide which E&M code to assign to a visit, it is important to know what is necessary to support the assigning of the code.

The E&M codes are based on seven components, but patient history, physical examination, and the complexity of the medical decision making are the key components. Those components are broken down by the extent of services provided in each of the major areas. For example, the extent of the history taken and the examination performed is a clinical judgment that may be seen as problem focused, expanded problem focused, detailed, or comprehensive.

CPT defines four types of medical decision making: straightforward, low complexity, moderate complexity, and high complexity. The level of coding and thus the reimbursement for services is determined by the mix of these key components.

In the introductory pages for E&M codes there is further detail to assist in understanding the key components. Also, the description of the services after the code lists the necessary components. For new patients, all three key components must be present and documented for any office service. For established patients, at least two key components must be present and documented. Additionally, Appendix C of the CPT book has clinical examples to help everyone understand how to select the correct code.

The remaining four components that are factored into determining the appropriate E&M code are nature of the presenting problem, counseling the patient or family member, length of the visit (time), and coordination of care with other providers. Pay particular attention to the introductory pages of the E&M section to gain a better understanding of how to code properly.

The next four sections of CPT are related to specific areas of medicine: anesthesia, surgery, radiology, and pathology/lab.

All anesthesia services are reported by the anatomical structure. For example, if the patient is having some kind of surgery on his or her knee, the anesthesiologist will use CPT codes from 01329 to 01444. Additionally, the anesthesiologist must report the physical status of the patient by a modifier. Modifiers are explained on page 143.

Surgery codes are also reported by anatomical structure. The rules are very specific about what is included in the surgical "package" so care must be taken not to code and bill separately for services that are considered part of the surgery. Most surgical packages include the office visit on or before the day of surgery, the operation itself, and normal follow-up care. These different components are bundled together in one single code. The introductory pages of the surgery section explain many of the restrictions. Medicare and many insurance companies have a set number of follow-up days for care after surgery. It is important to check for any restrictions before the procedure is done.

The radiology section of CPT is divided into four subsections: diagnostic radiology, diagnostic ultrasound, radiation oncology, and nuclear medicine. Within each subsection, the codes are generally arranged by anatomic site. Many of the codes indicate the number of views for a particular test. Some radiology procedures require a contrast medium be used. A contrast medium is the liquid administered to the patient before the procedure to enhance the images. If the contrast medium is given intravascularly, the proper code is the one that indicates with contrast. If the contrast medium is given orally or rectally, the proper code is the one that indicates without contrast.

The pathology and laboratory section of the CPT covers drug testing, panels of tests, chemistry testing, antibody testing, urinalysis, and consultations with pathologists. The first five areas cover almost every possible diagnostic lab test known. The last section, consultation with a pathologist, covers those services specifically provided by a pathologist. A pathologist is a medical doctor specifically trained in interpreting diagnostic tests.

The last section of the CPR is the Medicine section. This section has over 30 subsections that cover a wide variety of procedures. In the Medicine section you will find the CPT codes for vaccines, mental health counseling, chemotherapy administration, dermatology procedures, chiropractic manipulative treatments, and conscious sedation to mention only a few.

Table 9.1 shows the six areas of CPT coding. Even if you do not have responsibility for coding, you should become familiar with this important process.

The *Current Procedural Terminology,* Fourth Edition (CPT) is usually at least 900 pages long. How do you find the correct code? Understanding how to generally use CPT coding takes a little practice.

As mentioned, the book is divided into six sections. At the beginning of each section there is an explanation of the types of CPT codes found in that section. However, thumbing through the 900 pages trying to find the right code is probably not the easiest way to find the code.

**Table 9.1** CPT Coding Classification

- Evaluation and Management (99201–99499)
- Anesthesiology (00100–01999, 99100–99140)
- Surgery (10021–69990)
- Radiology (includes nuclear medicine and diagnostic ultrasound; 70010–79999)
- Pathology and Laboratory Services (80048–89356)
- Medicine (except Anesthesiology; 90281–99199, 99500–99902)

**Table 9.2** CPT Index Terms

- Procedure or service. For example: cholecystectomy, hysteroscopy.
- Organ or other anatomic site. For example: gall bladder, uterus.
- Condition. For example: cholelithiasis, uterine cancer.
- Synonyms, eponyms, and abbreviations. For example: EEG, ECS.

The alphabetic index located in the back of the book is your first step. This index is almost 200 pages long and is very detailed. It is organized alphabetically by four main types of terms, as shown in Table 9.2.

Using only the alphabetic index to determine a CPT code is not recommended. It is important to check the main text to determine if the code selected is appropriate. There are often subtle distinctions between two very similar procedures. Also, some CPT codes may need to be modified.

CPT codes may be modified under appropriate circumstances. Two-digit modifiers are used to give a more accurate description of the services provided. A modifier is used at the end of CPT code to indicate circumstances in which a procedure performed differed in some way from the standard description of the five-digit code. For example, two surgeons may be needed to manage a specific surgical problem that requires both surgeons working together as primary surgeons performing distinct parts of a procedure. In this case, both surgeons would modify the associated surgical procedure code with the modifier -92. You will find a complete list of modifiers in Appendix A of your *Current Procedural Terminology,* Fourth Edition (CPT).

Throughout the listing of procedures in the first six sections, you will see symbols in front of some codes. The Introduction section of the CPT manual provides some explanation. Additionally, the symbols' meanings are noted on the bottom of each page of the CPT book. For example, the plus sign (+) in front of a procedure means an add-on code. An add-on code is a supplemental service to another service performed by the same physician. The add-on code requires another code to be selected along with the + code. A second important symbol is the modifier -51 exempt Ø symbol. Often more than one procedure is performed for a patient during a single session. The additional procedures are modified with -51 unless they are exempt. An arrow with a circle around it ➔ is an important reminder for the coder to check the *CPT Assistant* newsletters or the annual *CPT Changes: An Insiders View* for further information. Information regarding these two important publications may be found in the Introduction of the CPT manual. This newsletter and annually revised book are important for staff members responsible for coding.

## Healthcare Common Procedure Coding System (HCPCS)

When seeking reimbursement for such items as medications, orthotics, or medical equipment, HCPCS Level II codes are used. The index for HCPCS codes is usually found in the front of the book as that is the first place to look for the appropriate code. HCPCS code books also have color coding to aid in determining whether the service is covered by Medicare or other third-party payers. The HCPCS Level II books often contain a variety of appendixes to assist in determining the proper code. Table 9.3 illustrates the main areas of HCPCS chapters.

**Table 9.3** HCPCS Chapter Headings

Chapter A Transportation Services Including Ambulance and Medical/Surgical Supplies

A0021–A0999 Transportation Services

A4000–A8999 Medical and Surgical Supplies

Chapter B Enteral and Parenteral Therapy (B4034–B9999)

Chapter C Outpatient Prospective Payment System (C1079–C9727)

These codes are to be used only in outpatient surgery centers.

Chapter D Dental Procedures (D0000–D9999)

Chapter E Durable Medical Equipment (E0100–E9999)

Chapter G Procedures/Professional Services (G0000–G9999)

Temporarily used in lieu of CPT codes.

Chapter H Alcohol and Drug Abuse Treatment Services (H0001–H2037)

The H codes are used by state Medicaid agencies that are mandated by state law to establish separate codes for identifying mental health services associated with alcohol and drug treatment.

Chapter J Drugs Administered Other than Oral Method (J0000–J9999)

Chapter K Temporary Codes (K0000–K9999)

Used in conjunction with durable medical equipment administrators contracted with Medicare and are often changed.

(*continued*)

Proper CPT coding is important. Improper codes could mean inappropriate or no reimbursement. More importantly, inappropriate CPT coding on insurance claims could lead to investigation by the CMS, possible loss of participation privileges, and even a felony conviction. Other third-party insurers also routinely audit claims, looking for what is called upcoding. **Upcoding** is when a provider submits a higher level code of service than was actually provided to obtain a higher reimbursement. **Downcoding** is when a provider submits a lower level code for a service that should have been coded at a higher level. Both are considered inappropriate and could lead to investigation and loss of participation. Fraud charges could also be filed.

Accurate CPT coding is critical for the success of the practice. Most practices have what is called an **encounter form** or superbill. On that form, the most commonly used CPT codes are listed. The provider may check or circle those codes that are most appropriate.

Depending on the sophistication of the office's billing software, it may be necessary to check for modifiers. Ultimately, the responsibility for the proper code lies with the provider of the services, but it is important that all staff have a basic understanding of CPT

**Table 9.3** HCPCS Chapter Headings (concluded)

| |
|---|
| Chapter L Orthotic Procedures and Devices (L0000–L4999) |
| Chapter M Medical Services (M0000–M0301) |
| These are mostly physician office services not listed elsewhere and are either obsolete services or services where their effect has not been proven. |
| Chapter P Pathology and Laboratory Services (P2028–P9615) |
| Chapter Q Temporary Codes (Q0000–Q9999) |
| Another miscellaneous section used by local contractors. |
| Chapter R Diagnostic Radiology Services (R0000–R5999) |
| R codes fall under the jurisdiction of the local contractors. |
| Chapter S Temporary National Codes (non-Medicare) (S0012–S0099) |
| S codes are used by Blue Cross/Blue Shield to report drugs and other services for which there are no national codes. Medicaid also uses these codes, but Medicare does not. |
| Chapter T Codes for State Medicaid Agencies (T1000–T9999) |
| Chapter V Vision Services (V2100–V5394) |
| V codes fall under the jurisdiction of the DME Medicare administrative contractor. |

**Table 9.4** Basic CPT Dos and Don'ts

| CPT Coding Steps |
|---|
| • Be certain you are using the latest edition of the CPT book. |
| • Even if you are a certified coder, don't make assumptions—check the guidelines and the *CPT Assistant* regularly. |
| • Make sure the diagnosis code (or codes) links to the CPT code. Never change the diagnosis code without consulting with the care provider. |
| • Ask the provider to clarify whenever necessary. Don't be afraid to ask. |
| • Routine audits to ensure proper documentation are a good idea. If CMS or a third-party payer questions a code, the appropriate documentation in the chart makes a big difference. |
| • Pay attention to CPT modifiers and use them appropriately. |

coding. Many offices have specific staff assigned to billing and coding. The American Medical Association (AMA) publishes the *CPT Assistant,* a newsletter written by CPT experts. The medical office should have at least one subscription to this newsletter. At the end of this chapter, you will find information about professional coding certifications.

Some suggested dos and don'ts for CPT may be found in Table 9.4. Training and education in the use of CPT coding are important—particularly for the staff members who do the actual coding.

## International Classification of Diseases, Ninth Revision

**International Classification of Diseases, Ninth Revision (ICD-9)** codes are the codes that identify the reason for the visit. These codes provide the diagnoses associated with the services provided. They are based on the official version of the World Health Organization's ninth revision of the *International Classification of Diseases.* The ICD-9-CM (International Classification of Diseases, Ninth Revision, Clinical Modification) classifies *morbidity* (illness) and *mortality* (death) information for statistical purposes.

The ICD-9-CM is updated every year in October. This update is done by four cooperating organizations: the American Hospital Association, the National Center for Health Statistics (NCHS), the Centers for Medicare and Medicaid Services (CMS), and the American Health Information Management Association (AHIMA).

As discussed previously, coding the diagnosis for each patient is very important. To do proper coding, you must have training in medical terminology. Some understanding of anatomy and physiology is also important.

In the outpatient setting, diagnoses must be coded based on the primary (first) diagnosis. The primary diagnosis is the main reason the patient came to see a physician or other health care provider. This could be a symptom such as vomiting, coughing, or diarrhea; an acute problem such as a laceration; or a chronic illness such as diabetes. Patients may often have more than one diagnosis, but it is critical to identify the primary diagnosis.

ICD-9 codes are usually five digits (numbers). However, ICD-9 codes may be three or four digits or may start with the letter *E* or *V*. M codes or morphology codes are used to further identify the behavior of a neoplasm and are used by cancer registries. M codes are not used when submitting claims to a third-party payer.

The ICD-9 code book consists of three volumes: Volume 1 is a tabular numerical listing of diagnosis codes; Volume 2 is the alphabetic listing of diagnoses; and Volume 3 is a combined tabular and alphabetic listing of procedures and is used primarily in the hospital setting. There are also five appendixes.

Volumes 1 and 2 are used by physicians and other care providers who are able to bill for their services. Like the CPT books it is important to get the update every year. Annual code changes are implemented on October 1.

Volume 2, the Index to Diseases, actually appears first in all ICD-9 books. That is because it is necessary to start with the index first to find the correct diagnostic code. There are three sections in Volume 2. Section One is the alphabetical listing of symptoms, signs, diagnoses, and conditions. Section Two is an alphabetic index to poisoning and external causes of adverse effects of drugs and other chemical substances. Section Three is an alphabetic index to external causes of injury.

Volume 1 lists all the diseases and injuries numerically. There are 17 chapters. Each chapter groups problems by cause (etiology) or anatomical site. See Table 9.5 for a complete list. Additionally, the V and E codes are listed, and there are several appendixes and tables at the end of Volume 1.

Each chapter is divided into sections of similar diseases. As an example, Chapter 7, Diseases of the Circulatory System, is divided into nine sections according to the type of disease that occurs in the circulatory system. Within each section, a three-digit code identifies the general disease category. If you look at the third disease section in the Chapter 7, you will see that it is hypertensive disease. Hypertensive disease is divided into five categories:

- 401 Essential hypertension
- 402 Hypertensive heart disease

**Table 9.5** ICD-9 Volume 1 Chapters, V and E Codes, Appendixes, and Tables

| Sections |
|---|
| Chapter 1—Infections and Parasitic Diseases (001–139) |
| Chapter 2—Neoplasms (140–239) |
| Chapter 3—Endocrine, Nutritional and Metabolic Immunity (240–279) |
| Chapter 4—Blood and Blood Forming Organs (280–289) |
| Chapter 5—Mental Disorders (290–319) |
| Chapter 9—Nervous System and Sense Organs (320–389) |
| Chapter 7—Diseases of the Circulatory System (390–459) |
| Chapter 8—Diseases of the Respiratory System (490–519) |
| Chapter 9—Diseases of the Digestive System (520–579) |
| Chapter 10—Genitourinary System (580–629) |
| Chapter 11—Complications of Pregnancy, Childbirth and the Puerperium (630–677) |
| Chapter 12—Skin and Subcutaneous Tissue (680–709) |
| Chapter 13—Diseases of the Musculoskeletal System and Connective Tissue (710–739) |
| Chapter 14—Congenital Anomalies (740–759) |
| Chapter 15—Certain Conditions Originating in the Perinatal Period (760–779) |
| Chapter 19—Symptoms, Signs and Ill-Defined Conditions (780–799) |
| Chapter 17—Injury and Poisoning (800–999) |
| **V and E Codes** |
| V Codes—Supplementary classification of factors influencing health status and contact with health services (V01–V83) |
| E Codes—Supplementary classification of external causes of injury and poisoning (E800–E999) |
| **Appendixes** |
| Appendix A—Morphology of Neoplasms |
| Appendix B—Glossary of Mental Disorders |
| Appendix C—Classification Drugs by AHFS List |
| Appendix D—Industrial Accidents According to Agency |
| Appendix E—List of Three-Digit Categories |

(continued)

**Table 9.5** ICD-9 Volume 1 Chapters, V and E Codes, Appendixes, and Tables (concluded)

| Tables |
|---|
| Valid three-digit code table |
| Abortion table |
| Burn table |
| Burn table—complications table |
| Diabetes table |
| Hernia table |
| Ectopic pregnancy table |
| Normal pregnancy table |
| Antepartum pregnancy table |
| Postpartum pregnancy table |

- 403 Hypertensive renal disease
- 404 Hypertensive heart and renal disease
- 405 Secondary hypertension

Within each disease category, a fourth and sometimes a fifth digit are necessary to identify the diagnosis correctly. These digits provide more specific information than just a three-digit code can and are placed after the first three digits. Here are two examples:

- 401.1 is benign essential hypertension.
- 404.11 is benign hypertensive heart and renal disease, without mention of heart failure or renal failure.

Care must be taken to include fourth and fifth digits where indicated in the ICD-9 code book. Failure to do so will mean nonpayment of the claim. Again, the example of essential hypertension illustrates the need for a fourth digit. Look at the code 401 in the ICD-9 code book. It will show a "check 4th digit" in front of the code. That means that unless a fourth digit is added, the coding is not correct. Professional coders will tell you that the first cardinal rule in coding is to code to the highest level of specificity when coding diagnoses.

As noted in Table 9.5, following the 17 chapters are the V codes and the E codes. V codes all begin with the letter *V.* These codes are used to identify patient encounters when the circumstances are other than an actual disease or injury. For example, there may be a personal or family history of disease, but the patient does not actually have that disease at the time of the visit. Or, the patient may have been exposed to an infectious disease, but has no symptoms. V codes are also used for immunizations and to code supervision of pregnancy. Table 9.6 contains a list of the major V code headings. V codes may be used as a primary diagnosis when appropriate.

V codes are separated into three main categories: problems, services, and factual findings. A problem is something that affects the patient's health status, such as a history of disease or a problem. For example, V12.52 is history of thrombophlebitis. This is not the primary diagnosis code, but would be important to record if the patient was being assessed for surgery. A service is when a patient is seen for something other than illness or injury. An example would be V09.1 which is the code for vaccination for diphtheria-tetanus-pertussis (DTP) with typhoid-parathyroid. Finally, factual findings are used to describe facts for statistical purposes. The most commonly used are codes related to reproduction and development. V33.01 is the code for twins delivered in the hospital by cesarean section.

Like the other diagnostic codes, V codes may have five digits. Using the V33.01 mentioned, the last two digits help specify the conditions. If the V code was V33.10, that would indicate that the twins (V33) were born before admission to the hospital (1) and without mention of cesarean section (0). As you can see, specificity is important.

The last area of diagnostic coding is E codes. These codes identify external causes of injury and poisoning and are used to code the events or circumstances surrounding the cause of injury, poisoning, or other adverse effect. For example, the patient may have been in a minor auto accident and comes to the office because his or her neck is strained. The

**Table 9.6** V Codes

| Codes | Description |
|---|---|
| V01–V06 | Persons with potential health hazards related to communicable diseases |
| V07–V09 | Persons with need for isolation, other potential health hazards and prophylactic measures |
| V10–V19 | Persons with potential health hazards related to personal and family history |
| V20–V28 | Persons encountering health services in circumstances related to personal and family history |
| V30–V39 | Healthy live born infants according to type of birth |
| V40–V49 | Persons with a condition influencing health status |
| V50–V59 | Persons encountering health services for specific procedures and after care |
| V60–V68 | Persons encountering health services in other circumstances |
| V70–V83 | Persons without reported diagnosis encountering during examination and investigation of individuals and population |

diagnostic code for the neck strain is 847.0. However, it will be important to code for the circumstances (auto accident) also. E codes are never used alone. They are always at least secondary to the primary diagnosis.

Why is it important to do E coding? There may be many different payers involved in a patient's care, particularly if the care is needed because of an accident. In the previous example, auto insurance (either the patient's or the person's who caused the accident) is responsible for payment of the costs associated with care. The patient's primary health insurance is not liable for any costs until the limits on the auto insurance liability have been exhausted. Even then, there may be problems with coverage. E coding assists the payers in sorting out who is responsible. Table 9.7 illustrates some of the major E codes.

Diagnostic coding is complicated. To appropriately code an office visit or other outpatient procedure, there are steps that should be followed routinely. Keep in mind that if an incorrect or inappropriate code is submitted for billing, not only may the practice not be paid, but you may be inadvertently labeling a patient with an illness he or she does not have. The second cardinal rule in ICD-9 in the outpatient setting is that you code signs and symptoms if you do not have a confirmed diagnosis. Fever, headache, muscle and joint ache, sore throat, and diarrhea are all symptoms of HIV, but they are also symptoms of the flu. In a case like this, the medical professional who may suspect HIV will be sure to get a detailed patient history looking for known risk behaviors that could lead to HIV. For purposes of coding the first visit, the signs and symptom already mentioned would be coded, not HIV. Table 9.8 provides you with a list of those steps.

That same encounter form or superbill discussed earlier is used by the provider to indicate a diagnosis. However, there are thousands of diagnoses, so only those most commonly found in your specialty are likely to be listed on the encounter form or superbill. If the diagnosis is not listed, the provider can write it on the form. Then the checkout staff must use the ICD-9 book to code the diagnosis to be entered into the billing system.

You will need to go through this same process for each sign, symptom, diagnosis, or condition. Be sure that the first code listed is the primary diagnosis. Do not code conditions when the provider has said "suspected," "rule out," "questionable," or "probable." As mentioned, the symptoms are coded. Until you have a confirmed diagnosis, you cannot code a disease.

Most offices use a computer system to enter both CPT and ICD-9 codes. The primary diagnosis must be identified and, as discussed, CPT and the ICD-9 codes must be linked. Individual software packages differ, but it is critical that attention is paid to identifying the primary diagnosis, as well as linking CPT and ICD-9 codes. For example, a patient comes in for her annual physical exam. A part of her annual exam is a mammogram as well as other screening tests done in the office. The patient may complain of a rapid heartbeat.

## Table 9.7 Major E Codes

| | |
|---|---|
| E800–E807 | Railway accidents |
| E810–E819 | Motor vehicle accidents |
| E820–E825 | Vehicle nontraffic accidents |
| E825–E829 | Other road vehicle accidents |
| E830–E838 | Water transport accidents |
| E840–E845 | Air and space transport accidents |
| E849–E848 | Vehicle accidents not elsewhere classifiable |
| E849 | Category used to identify the place of occurrence for E800–E848 |
| E850–E858 | Accidental poisoning by drugs, medicinal substances and biologicals |
| E860–E869 | Accidental poisoning by other solid and liquid substances, gases and vapors |
| E870–E879 | Misadventures to patients during surgical and medical care |
| E879–E879 | Surgical and medical procedures as the cause of abnormal reaction of patient or later complication, without mention of misadventure at the time of procedure |
| E880–E888 | Accidental falls |
| E890–E899 | Accidents caused by fire and flames |
| E900–E909 | Accidents due to natural and environmental factors |
| E910–E915 | Accidents caused by submersion, suffocation and foreign bodies |
| E916–E928 | Other accidents |
| E930–E949 | Drugs, medicinal and biological substances causing adverse effects in therapeutic use |
| E950–E959 | Suicide and self-inflicted injury |
| E960–E969 | Homicide and injury purposely inflicted by other persons |
| E970–E978 | Legal intervention |
| E979 | Terrorism |
| E980–E989 | Injury undetermined whether accidentally or purposely inflicted |
| E990–E999 | Injury resulting from operations of war |

*Note:* At the beginning of the chapter on E codes there are specific instructions regarding the coding of accidents involving vehicles with a motor.

Table 9.8 ICD-9 Coding Steps

1. Identify the reason for the visit—the sign, symptom, diagnosis, or condition.
2. Look up the main term or disease in the alphabetic index (Volume 2). The main term is what is wrong with the patient and is printed in bold in Volume 2. Examples of main terms are *abnormal, allergy, deficiency fracture, sprain,* and so on. Also, the name of the disease or condition *(deafness, diarrhea, diabetes, myocarditis)* is a main term and is used to find the area to check in Volume 1. *Never* code by simply using the code found in the alphabetic index.
3. Identify the subterms. Below the main terms are subterms that further describe the main terms. For example, under the disease Diabetes, there are over 100 subterms.
4. Choose a code and locate it in Volume 1, the numerical list.
5. Determine if the code you have selected is at the highest level of specificity. In other words, select the three-digit code only if there are no four- or five-digit codes within that code category. Five-digit coding should always be used when available. Most ICD-9 code books have a small box or circle to the left of the main term that will say "Check 4th digit" or "Check 5th digit."
6. Assign the code.

The physician does not yet know what the cause of the rapid heartbeat is. The physician may have an EKG done in the office the same day the mammogram is done. The symptom tachycardia (fast heartbeat) would be linked to the EKG procedure code and not linked to the CPT code for mammography.

## International Classification of Diseases, Tenth Revision

The talk about implementing International Classification of Diseases, Tenth Revision (ICD-10) for general use in the United States has been ongoing since the mid-nineties. As of the publication date of this book, the only use of ICD-10 is to code and classify mortality dates from death certificates. In July 2007 a new release of ICD-10-CM (International Classification of Diseases, Tenth Revision, Clinical Modification) was made available for public viewing. However, the codes in ICD-10-CM are not currently valid for any purpose or use and no comments are being sought on the content of ICD-10. Furthermore, there is not yet an anticipated implementation date for the ICD-10-CM. Check the National Center for Health Statistics website for further updates.

## Professional Coders

Although it may seem that with some practice, it might be a somewhat simple process to do both CPT and ICD-9 coding, that is not the case. A good knowledge of medical terminology, anatomy, and physiology is necessary. A thorough knowledge of rules and regulations regarding coding is critical. Certified coders are in demand throughout the country. If you are interested in becoming a certified professional coder, contact either the American Academy of Professional Coders (AAPC) or the American Health Information Management Association (AHIMA). All of the certified coders must take and pass a national exam, as well as maintain continuing education units (CEUs) after successfully completing the exam. There are various other requirements for these certifications, so it is important to contact the organization directly. The various types of coder certifications are found in Table 9.9.

**Table 9.9** Coding Certification Levels

| American Health Information Management Association (AHIMA) |
|---|
| RHIA—Registered Health Information Administrator: skilled in collection, interpretation, and analysis of medical data; usually are management positions; must possess a bachelor's degree from an accredited institution. |
| RHIT—Registered Health Information Technician: midlevel coder who also may do data analysis. |
| CCS—Certified Coding Specialist: midlevel hospital-focused coder. |
| CCS-P—Certified Coding Specialist–Physician-based: midlevel physician-based coder. |
| CCA—Certified Coding Associate: entry-level coder. |
| **American Academy of Professional Coders (AAPC)** |
| CPC—Certified professional coder for physician services. |
| CPC-H—Certified professional coder for outpatient/facility services. |
| CPC-P—Certified professional coder for payer. |
| AAPC also awards an apprentice certification for these three levels of certification for individuals who are successful in passing the certification examination, but have not met the required 2 years of coding work experience. Once the individual has documented 2 years of work experience, provided evidence of 39 CEUs every 2 years, and maintained continual membership in the AAPC, the individual receives the official AAPC CPC, CPC-H, or CPC-P diploma. |

## Summary

Coding is an important aspect of the health care business. Coding is the translation of procedures, services, supplies, and diagnoses into numeric and sometimes alphanumeric codes for reimbursement and statistical purposes. The HCPCS contains Level I (CPT) codes and Level II (HCPCS) codes to identify procedures, services, and supplies provided to the patient. ICD-9 codes are used to identify diagnoses. Medical coding is a complex process requiring knowledge of medical terminology, anatomy, and physiology. Certified coders can help prevent legal difficulties and ensure that providers receive full reimbursement in a timely manner. The rules for coding are established by the Centers for Medicare and Medicaid Services and the World Health Organization. Insurance companies also use these codes. Proper coding provides important information not only to third-party payers, but to the nation as well.

# Chapter 10

# The Daily Business in the Medical Office—Accounting and Bookkeeping

## Introduction

*As you are probably already aware, the financial side of health care is a confusing one. With so many different kinds of health care organizations and ways for a patient's bill to be paid, it is difficult to keep it all straight. Chapter 8 covered the various types of health insurance. Because much of the money collected comes from a third-party payer, not the patient, it is sometimes difficult to understand the individual patient's account. Since the staff is usually responsible for explaining to the patient the balance due or how the third-party payment works, it is important that all office staff members have a basic understanding of how the accounting and bookkeeping system works.*

*Most medical offices use computerized systems to enter charges and payments, generate receipts, and create bills to be mailed or electronically submitted. As we discussed in Chapter 4, a computerized system, often called a practice management system (PMS), is very important in generating the information necessary for the prescribed billing forms. Much of the billing to insurance companies is now done electronically. Medicare requires electronic billing. To aid in your understanding of the system, this chapter provides a description of the process from the beginning, when the new patient is first seen, to the end, when the patient has a zero balance.*

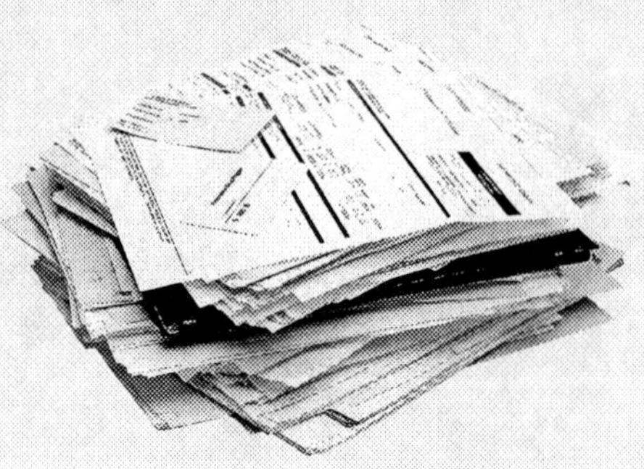

## Chapter Outline

## Processing a New Patient

**Step 1.** The new patient arrives for the first visit. It is necessary to set up an **account** for him or her. This account will be part of the **accounting** system that tracks all financial information for the practice.

It is important to collect information from the patient on a patient registration form, sometimes called a patient data sheet. A variety of demographic and health information is collected before the patient is seen. Let's focus on the demographic information.

The patient registration form collects all the important information you need to know to determine how the patient is going to pay the bill. It also provides pertinent information about where the patient works, telephone numbers, and who to contact in an emergency. Figure 10.1 shows a sample patient registration form.

Many practices have the patient complete the patient registration form (along with other forms to be discussed) before the day of the visit. The practice can either mail the forms to the patient or, as is increasingly done, ask the patient to go the practice's website to download them. If your practice has patients fill out the forms when they come into the office for the first visit, be sure to have them come in at least 15 minutes early. When making the appointment, remind them to bring their insurance cards with them as well.

Each medical practice should inform the new patient of his or her financial policies and have the patient sign an acknowledgment that the policies are understood. Figure 10.2 illustrates a sample financial policy. Although each medical specialty differs somewhat, the patient should also fill out a health history form. A sample is shown in Figure 10.3.

Most practices now require a form of picture identification, usually a driver's license or other identification card. This is done to prevent the fraudulent use of health insurance benefits.

Depending on your practice, it may be necessary to counsel the new patient before he or she is seen by the health care provider. If the practice does not participate in certain insurance plans, or offers elective services usually not covered by various health insurance or Medicare, the patient must be made aware of this *before* being seen by the

Jones Family Practice
1023 Pontiac Drive
Hillsborough, Ohio 34567

Welcome to our practice. We need to collect some basic information from you today.

Last name _______________ First name _________ MI _____
Birth date _______ Sex _____ Age _____
Local address ____________ City _______ Zip ___

For patients who are retired, you will need to add lines for alternate address, city, state, zip, and phone number.

Local phone number _______ Work phone _______ Cell phone ______
Email address _______
Employer _______Occupation _______
Employer address _______ City _______ State _______ Zip _____

For specialty practices, you will need to add lines for the patient to indicate who his or her primary care physician is.

Person legally responsible for this account _______ self _______ other—please complete the following:

Name _______ Relationship to patient _______
Birth date _______ Sex ___
Address _______ City _______State ___ Zip ___
Home phone _______ Work phone _______

In an emergency, please contact _______ at _______.

Please provide your driver's license and your insurance cards to the receptionist.

I authorize the release of any medical or other information necessary to process this claim. I also assign to (Name of Practice) any insurance or other third-party benefits available for health care services provided to me by the (Name of Practice). If benefits are not assigned to (Name of Practice), I agree to forward to (Name of Practice) all health insurance and other third-party payments I may receive for services. These payments will be forwarded immediately upon receipt.

________________________________________ _____
Patient's or Patient's Representative's Signature Date

________________________________________
Print Patient's or Patient's Representative's Name

**Figure 10.1** Patient Registration Form

At ________ (Name of Practice), we are dedicated to providing the best possible care while maintaining your privacy. This does require that you understand our financial policies as part of your care and treatment. After reading this, if you have questions, do not hesitate to discuss our financial policy with our front office (or financial counselor if your office has one).

We are a participating provider with Medicare. We will bill Medicare for you. You are responsible for your annual deductible, copayments, and charges for noncovered services. You will be asked to sign an Advance Beneficiary Notice of Noncoverage for those services that we know are not covered by Medicare. You will need to pay for those services at the time they are provided, unless other arrangements are made.

Your insurance policy is a contract between you and your insurance company. We are a participating provider in a number of national health insurance plans. We will bill those plans that we participate in. You are expected to cover your deductible and copayments and noncovered services. We will make every effort to inform you of services that may not be covered, but each insurance company is different and the covered procedures do change. In the event your insurance company denies a claim for noncovered services, you will be billed after we receive that denial. Payment is expected in 30 days unless other arrangements are made.

We have agreements with a variety of plans and for those plans, we accept assignment of benefits. We bill those plans and require you to pay only the copayment, coinsurance, or deductible at the time of service. Covered services frequently change. We file your insurance as a courtesy to you. In the event that coverage is denied, you will be billed for the services provided.

Certain surgical procedures require prepayment and/or preauthorization. You will meet with a member of our staff to discuss this process. Payment will be due one week in advance of elective surgery.

It is your responsibility to inform us of all insurance changes and referral requirements. If we do not receive that information from you, you will be responsible for any charges.

Past due accounts are subject to collection, including the filing of a medical lien. We are willing to work with patients to establish a payment plan in the event of a large balance; however, that decision is at our discretion.

For those patients who have insurance coverage with a plan we do not participate in, we will prepare and send the claim for you on an unassigned basis. The insurance company will send the payment directly to you. Therefore, all charges for your care and treatment are due at the time of service. If the charges exceed $500, you will be asked to pay a

**Figure 10.2** Financial Policy Form (continued)

minimum of 50%, with the balance due in 45 days. This 45-day period allows time for the insurance company to pay you. If we do not have a contract with your plan, we are not obligated to adjust our charges based on your plan's benefit schedule or coverage.

If you have any questions regarding our financial policies, do not hesitate to discuss them with a member of our staff before you are seen as a patient.

I have read and understand the financial policies above:

Patient's or Patient's Representative's Signature Date

Print Patient's or Patient's Representative's Name

**Figure 10.2** (concluded)



provider. A copy of the 2008 Advance Beneficiary Notice of Noncoverage (ABN) required by Medicare is found in Figure 10.4.

**Step 2.** The new patient's information is entered into the practice management system (PMS).

Most practices have a computerized PMS. The front desk staff enter the demographic information about the patient into the system. It is important that the individuals entering the data carefully proof the information afterward. An incorrect policy or group number, address, or telephone number could create problems later on. Make a copy of both sides of the insurance card, and return the card to the patient. The patient registration form and copy of the insurance card go into the patient's chart.

Depending on your practice, insurance verification may need to be obtained before the patient is seen by the provider. This is done in one of two ways—calling the insurance company or entering a secure website of the insurance company to verify coverage.

Depending on the system used, either a computer-generated or hand-generated encounter form is created and put on top of the patient's newly created medical record folder. A sample encounter form is found in Figure 10.5. The chart and encounter form are then provided to the medical assistant or nurse who will take the patient to the exam room area to obtain further medical information.

**Step 3.** Depending on the type of practice, after the new patient has seen the provider but before he or she leaves the office, the patient is escorted to the checkout area

## HEALTH HISTORY
(Confidential)

Name__________ Today's Date__________

Age______ Birthdate__________ Date of last physical examination__________

What is your reason for visit?__________

**SYMPTOMS** Check (✓) symptoms you currently have or have had in the past year.

**GENERAL**
- ☐ Chills
- ☐ Depression
- ☐ Dizziness
- ☐ Fainting
- ☐ Fever
- ☐ Forgetfulness
- ☐ Headache
- ☐ Loss of sleep
- ☐ Loss of weight
- ☐ Nervousness
- ☐ Numbness
- ☐ Sweats

**MUSCLE/JOINT/BONE**
Pain, weakness, numbness in:
- ☐ Arms ☐ Hips
- ☐ Back ☐ Legs
- ☐ Feet ☐ Neck
- ☐ Hands ☐ Shoulders

**GENITO-URINARY**
- ☐ Blood in urine
- ☐ Frequent urination
- ☐ Lack of bladder control
- ☐ Painful urination

**GASTROINTESTINAL**
- ☐ Appetite poor
- ☐ Bloating
- ☐ Bowel changes
- ☐ Constipation
- ☐ Diarrhea
- ☐ Excessive hunger
- ☐ Excessive thirst
- ☐ Gas
- ☐ Hemorrhoids
- ☐ Indigestion
- ☐ Nausea
- ☐ Rectal bleeding
- ☐ Stomach pain
- ☐ Vomiting
- ☐ Vomiting blood

**CARDIOVASCULAR**
- ☐ Chest pain
- ☐ High blood pressure
- ☐ Irregular heart beat
- ☐ Low blood pressure
- ☐ Poor circulation
- ☐ Rapid heart beat
- ☐ Swelling of ankles
- ☐ Varicose veins

**EYE, EAR, NOSE, THROAT**
- ☐ Bleeding gums
- ☐ Blurred vision
- ☐ Crossed eyes
- ☐ Difficulty swallowing
- ☐ Double vision
- ☐ Earache
- ☐ Ear discharge
- ☐ Hay fever
- ☐ Hoarseness
- ☐ Loss of hearing
- ☐ Nosebleeds
- ☐ Persistent cough
- ☐ Ringing in ears
- ☐ Sinus problems
- ☐ Vision – Flashes
- ☐ Vision – Halos

**SKIN**
- ☐ Bruise easily
- ☐ Hives
- ☐ Itching
- ☐ Change in moles
- ☐ Rash
- ☐ Scars
- ☐ Sore that won't heal

**MEN only**
- ☐ Breast lump
- ☐ Erection difficulties
- ☐ Lump in testicles
- ☐ Penis discharge
- ☐ Sore on penis
- ☐ Other

**WOMEN only**
- ☐ Abnormal Pap smear
- ☐ Bleeding between periods
- ☐ Breast lump
- ☐ Extreme menstrual pain
- ☐ Hot flashes
- ☐ Nipple discharge
- ☐ Painful intercourse
- ☐ Vaginal discharge
- ☐ Other

Date of last menstrual period______

Date of last Pap smear______

Have you had a mammogram?______

Are you pregnant?______

Number of children______

**CONDITIONS** Check (✓) conditions you have or have had in the past.

- ☐ AIDS
- ☐ Alcoholism
- ☐ Anemia
- ☐ Anorexia
- ☐ Appendicitis
- ☐ Arthritis
- ☐ Asthma
- ☐ Bleeding Disorders
- ☐ Breast Lump
- ☐ Bronchitis
- ☐ Bulimia
- ☐ Cancer
- ☐ Cataracts
- ☐ Chemical Dependency
- ☐ Chicken Pox
- ☐ Diabetes
- ☐ Emphysema
- ☐ Epilepsy
- ☐ Glaucoma
- ☐ Goiter
- ☐ Gonorrhea
- ☐ Gout
- ☐ Heart Disease
- ☐ Hepatitis
- ☐ Hernia
- ☐ Herpes
- ☐ High Cholesterol
- ☐ HIV Positive
- ☐ Kidney Disease
- ☐ Liver Disease
- ☐ Measles
- ☐ Migraine Headaches
- ☐ Miscarriage
- ☐ Mononucleosis
- ☐ Multiple Sclerosis
- ☐ Mumps
- ☐ Pacemaker
- ☐ Pneumonia
- ☐ Polio
- ☐ Prostate Problem
- ☐ Psychiatric Care
- ☐ Rheumatic Fever
- ☐ Scarlet Fever
- ☐ Stroke
- ☐ Suicide Attempt
- ☐ Thyroid Problems
- ☐ Tonsillitis
- ☐ Tuberculosis
- ☐ Typhoid Fever
- ☐ Ulcers
- ☐ Vaginal Infections
- ☐ Venereal Disease

| **MEDICATIONS** List medications you are currently taking | **ALLERGIES** To medications or substances |
|---|---|
| | |
| | |
| | |
| | |
| Pharmacy Name______ Phone______ | |

Figure 10.3 Health History Form (continued)

Source: Booth et al., *Medical Assisting*, 3e, p. 709. Copyright © 2005 The McGraw-Hill Companies, Inc. Reprinted with permission.

**(All information is strictly confidential)**

**FAMILY HISTORY** Fill in health information about your family.

| Relation | Age | State of Health | Age at Death | Cause of Death |
|---|---|---|---|---|
| Father | | | | |
| Mother | | | | |
| Brothers | | | | |
| | | | | |
| | | | | |
| | | | | |
| Sisters | | | | |
| | | | | |
| | | | | |
| | | | | |

**Check (✓) if your blood relatives had any of the following:**

| ✓ | Disease | Relationship to you |
|---|---|---|
| | Arthritis, Gout | |
| | Asthma, Hay Fever | |
| | Cancer | |
| | Chemical Dependency | |
| | Diabetes | |
| | Heart Disease, Strokes | |
| | High Blood Pressure | |
| | Kidney Disease | |
| | Tuberculosis | |
| | Other | |

**HOSPITALIZATIONS**

| Year | Hospital | Reason for Hospitalization and Outcome |
|---|---|---|
| | | |
| | | |
| | | |
| | | |
| | | |
| | | |
| | | |
| | | |
| | | |
| | | |

**PREGNANCY HISTORY**

| Year of Birth | Sex of Birth | Complications if any |
|---|---|---|
| | | |
| | | |
| | | |
| | | |
| | | |
| | | |
| | | |

**HEALTH HABITS** Check (✓) which substances you use and describe how much you use.

| ✓ | Substance | Amount |
|---|---|---|
| | Caffeine | |
| | Tobacco | |
| | Drugs | |
| | Other | |
| | | |

**Have you ever had a blood transfusion?** ☐ Yes ☐ No
If yes, please give approximate dates.________

| SERIOUS ILLNESS/INJURIES | DATE | OUTCOME |
|---|---|---|
| | | |
| | | |
| | | |
| | | |
| | | |
| | | |
| | | |
| | | |
| | | |
| | | |

**OCCUPATIONAL CONCERNS**
Check (✓) if your work exposes you to the following:

| | |
|---|---|
| | Stress |
| | Hazardous Substances |
| | Heavy Lifting |
| | Other |

Your occupation:

I certify that the above information is correct to the best of my knowledge. I will not hold my doctor or any members of his/her staff responsible for any errors or omissions that I may have made in the completion of this form.

________________ Signature ________________ Date

________________ Reviewed By ________________ Date

**Figure 10.3** (concluded)

**(*A*) Notifier(s):**

**(*B*) Patient Name:** **(*C*) Identification Number:**

## ADVANCE BENEFICIARY NOTICE OF NONCOVERAGE (ABN)

***NOTE:*** If Medicare doesn't pay for ***(D)***_________________ below, you may have to pay.

Medicare does not pay for everything, even some care that you or your health care provider have good reason to think you need. We expect Medicare may not pay for the ***(D)***____________ below.

| *(D)*_____________ | *(E)* Reason Medicare May Not Pay | *(F)* Estimated Cost |
|---|---|---|
| | | |

**WHAT YOU NEED TO DO NOW:**

- Read this notice, so you can make an informed decision about your care.
- Ask us any questions that you may have after you finish reading.
- Choose an option below about whether to receive the ***(D)***____________ listed above.

  **Note:** If you choose Option 1or 2, we may help you to use any other insurance that you might have, but Medicare cannot require us to do this.

| ***(G)* Options:** Check only one box: We cannot choose a box for you |
|---|
| ☐ **OPTION 1.** I want the ***(D)*** __________ listed above. You may ask to be paid now, but I also want Medicare billed for an official decision on payment, which is sent to me on a Medicare Summary Notice (MSN). I understand that if Medicare doesn't pay, I am responsible for payment, but **I can appeal to Medicare** by following the directions on the MSN. If Medicare does pay, you will refund any payments I made to you, less co-pays or deductibles. |
| ☐ **OPTION 2.** I want the ***(D)*** __________ listed above, but do not bill Medicare. You may ask to be paid now as I am responsible for payment. **I cannot appeal if Medicare is not billed.** |
| ☐ **OPTION 3.** I don't want the ***(D)*** __________ listed above. I understand with this choice I am **not** responsible for payment, and **I cannot appeal to see if Medicare would pay.** |

***(H)* Additional Information:**

**This notice gives our opinion, not an official Medicare decision.** If you have other questions on this notice or Medicare billing, call **1-800-MEDICARE** (1-800-633-4227/**TTY**: 1-877-486-2048). Signing below means that you have received and understand this notice. You also receive a copy.

| ***(I)* Signature:** | ***(J)* Date:** |
|---|---|

According to the Paperwork Reduction Act of 1995, no persons are required to respond to a collection of information unless it displays a valid OMB control number. The valid OMB control number for this information collection is 0938-0566. The time required to complete this information collection is estimated to average 7 minutes per response, including the time to review instructions, search existing data resources gather the data needed, and complete and review the information collectiion. If you have comments concerning accuracy of the time estimate or suggestions for improving this form, please with in CMS 7500 Security Boulevard. Attn: PEA Repons Clearance Officer, Baltimore, Maryland 21204-1850.

Form CMS-R-131 (03/08) Form Approved OMB No. 0938-0566

**Figure 10.4** Advance Beneficiary Notice of Noncoverage (ABN)

Source: www.cms.hhs.gov/BNI/02_ABNGABNL.asp.

*Lakeridge Medical Group*
*262 East Pine Street, Suite 100*
*Santa Cruz, CA 95062*

☐ PRIVATE ☐ BLUECROSS ☐ IND. ☐ MEDICARE ☐ MEDI-CAL ☐ HMO ☐ PPO

| PATIENT'S LAST NAME | FIRST | ACCOUNT # | BIRTHDATE / / | SEX ☐ MALE ☐ FEMALE | TODAY'S DATE / / |
|---|---|---|---|---|---|
| INSURANCE COMPANY | SUBSCRIBER | | PLAN # | SUB. # | GROUP |

ASSIGNMENT: I hereby assign my insurance benefits to be paid directly to the undersigned physician. I am financially responsible for non-covered services. SIGNED: (Patient, or Parent, if Minor) DATE: / /

RELEASE: I hereby authorize the physician to release to my insurance carrers any information required to process this claim. SIGNED: (Patient, or Parent, if Minor) DATE: / /

| ✓ | DESCRIPTION | M/Care | CPT/Mod | DxRe | FEE |
|---|---|---|---|---|---|
| | OFFICE CARE | | | | |
| | NEW PATIENT | | | | |
| | Brief | | 99201 | | |
| | Limited | | 99202 | | |
| | Intermediate | | 99203 | | |
| | Extended | | 99204 | | |
| | Comprehensive | | 99205 | | |
| | | | | | |
| | ESTABLISHED PATIENT | | | | |
| | Minimal | | 99211 | | |
| | Brief | | 99212 | | |
| | Limited | | 99213 | | |
| | Intermediate | | 99214 | | |
| | Extended | | 99215 | | |
| | Comprehensive | | 99215 | | |
| | | | | | |
| | CONSULTATION-OFFICE | | | | |
| | Focused | | 99241 | | |
| | Expanded | | 99242 | | |
| | Detailed | | 99243 | | |
| | Comprehensive 1 | | 99244 | | |
| | Comprehensive 2 | | 99245 | | |
| | Dr. | | | | |
| | Case Management | | 98900 | | |
| | | | | | |
| | Post-op Exam | | 99024 | | |
| | | | | | |
| | | | | | |
| | | | | | |

| ✓ | DESCRIPTION | M/Care | CPT/Mod | DxRe | FEE |
|---|---|---|---|---|---|
| | PROCEDURES | | | | |
| | Tread Mill (In Office) | | 93015 | | |
| | 24 Hour Holter | | 93224 | | |
| | If Medicare (Set up Fec) | | 93225 | | |
| | Physician Interpret | | 93227 | | |
| | EKG w/Interpretation | | 93000 | | |
| | EKG (Medicare) | | 93005 | | |
| | Sigmoidoscopy | | 45300 | | |
| | Sigmoidoscopy, Flexible | | 45330 | | |
| | Sigmoidos. , Flex. w/Bx. | | 45331 | | |
| | Spirometry, FEV/FVC | | 94010 | | |
| | Spirometry, Post-Dilator | | 94060 | | |
| | | | | | |
| | | | | | |
| | LABORATORY | | | | |
| | Blood Draw Fee | | 36415 | | |
| | Urinalysis, Chemical | | 81005 | | |
| | Throat Culture | | 87081 | | |
| | Occult Blood | | 82270 | | |
| | Pap Handling Charge | | 99000 | | |
| | Pap Life Guard | | 88150-90 | | |
| | Gram Stain | | 87205 | | |
| | Hanging Drop | | 87210 | | |
| | Urine Drug Screen | | 99000 | | |
| | | | | | |
| | | | | | |
| | SUPPLIES | | | | |
| | | | | | |
| | | | | | |
| | | | | | |

| ✓ | DESCRIPTION | M/Care | CPT/Mod | DxRe | FEE |
|---|---|---|---|---|---|
| | INJECTIONS/IMMUNIZATIONS | | | | |
| | Tetanus | | 90718 | | |
| | Hypertet | J1670 | 90782 | | |
| | Pneumococcal | | 90732 | | |
| | Influenza | | 90724 | | |
| | TB Skin Test (PPD) | | 86585 | | |
| | Antigen Injection-Single | | 95115 | | |
| | Multiple | | 95117 | | |
| | B12 Injection | J3420 | 90782 | | |
| | Injection, IM | | 90782 | | |
| | Compazine | J0780 | 90782 | | |
| | Demerol | J2175 | 90782 | | |
| | Vistaril | J3410 | 90782 | | |
| | Susphrine | J0170 | 90782 | | |
| | Decadron | J0890 | 90782 | | |
| | Estradiol | J1000 | 90782 | | |
| | Testosterone | J1080 | 90782 | | |
| | Lidocaine | J2000 | 90782 | | |
| | Solumedrol | J2920 | 90782 | | |
| | Solucortef | J1720 | 90782 | | |
| | Hydeltra | J1690 | 90782 | | |
| | Pen Procaine | J2510 | 90788 | | |
| | | | | | |
| | INJECTIONS - JOINT/BURSA | | | | |
| | Small Joints | | 20600 | | |
| | Intermediate | | 20605 | | |
| | Large Joints | | 20610 | | |
| | Trigger Point | | 20550 | | |
| | MISCELLANEOUS | | | | |
| | | | | | |

| DIAGNOSIS: | ICD-9 | | | | | | | | |
|---|---|---|---|---|---|---|---|---|---|
| ___ Abdominal Pain | 789.0 | ___ Gout | 274.0 | ___ C.V.A. - Acute | 436. | ___ Electrolyte Dis. | 276.9 | ___ Herpes Simplex | 054.9 |
| ___ Abscess (Site) | 682.9 | ___ Asthma | 493.90 | ___ Cere. Vas. Accid. (Old) | 438 | ___ Fatigue | 780.7 | ___ Herpes Zoster | 053.9 |
| ___ Adverse Drug Rx | 995.2 | ___ Asthmatic Bronchitis | 493.90 | ___ Cerumen | 380.4 | ___ Fibrocys. Br. Dis | 610.1 | ___ Hydrocele | 603.9 |
| ___ Alcohol Detox | 291.8 | ___ Atrial Fib. | 427.31 | ___ Chestwall Pain | 786.59 | ___ Fracture (Site) | 829.0 | ___ Hyperlipidemia | 272.4 |
| ___ Alcoholism | 303.90 | ___ Atrial Tachi. | 427.0 | ___ Cholecystitis | 575.0 | ___ Open/Close | | ___ Hypertension | 401.9 |
| ___ Allergic Rhinitis | 477 | ___ Bowel Obstruct. | 560.9 | ___ Cholelithiasis | 574.00 | ___ Fungal Infect. (Site) | 110.8 | ___ Hyperthyroidism | 242.9 |
| ___ Allergy | 995.3 | ___ Breast Mass | 611.72 | ___ COPD | 492.8 | ___ Gastric Ulcer | 531.90 | ___ Hypothyroidism | 244.9 |
| ___ Alzheimer's Dis. | 290.1 | ___ Bronchitis | 490 | ___ Cirrhosis | 571.5 | ___ Gastritis | 535.0 | ___ Labyrinthitis | 386.30 |
| ___ Anemia | 285.9 | ___ Bursitis | 727.3 | ___ Cong. Heart Fail. | 428.9 | ___ Gastroenteritis | 558.9 | ___ Lipoma (Site) | 214.9 |
| ___ Anemia - Pernicious | 281.0 | ___ Cancer, Breast (Site) | 174.9 | ___ Conjunctivitis | 372.30 | ___ G.I. Bleeding | 578.9 | ___ Lymphoma | 202.8 |
| ___ Angina | 413.9 | ___ Metastatic (Site) | 199.1 | ___ Contusion (Site) | 924.9 | ___ Glomerulonephritis | 583.9 | ___ Mit. Valve Prolapse | 424.0 |
| ___ Anxiety Synd. | 300.00 | ___ Colon | 153.9 | ___ Costochondritis | 733.99 | ___ Headache | 784.0 | ___ Myocard. Infarction (Area) | 410.9 |
| ___ Appendicitis | 541 | ___ Cancer, Rectal | 154.1 | ___ Depression | 311. | ___ Headache, Tension | 307.81 | ___ M.I., Old | 412 |
| ___ Arterioscl. H.D. | 414.0 | ___ Lung (Site) | 162.9 | ___ Dermatitis | 692.9 | ___ Migraine (Type) | 346.9 | ___ Myositis | 729.1 |
| ___ Arthritis, Osteo. | 715.90 | ___ Skin (Site) | 173.9 | ___ Diabetes Mellitus | 250.00 | ___ Hemorrhoids | 455.6 | ___ Nausea/Vomiting | 787.0 |
| ___ Rheumatoid | 714.0 | ___ Card. Arrhythmia (Type) | 427.9 | ___ Diabetic Ketosis | 250.1 | ___ Hernia, Hiatal | 553.3 | ___ Neuralgia | 729.2 |
| ___ Lupus | 710.0 | ___ Cardiomyopathy | 425.4 | ___ Diverticulitis | 562.11 | ___ Inguinal | 550.9 | ___ Nevus (Site) | 216.9 |
| | | ___ Cellulitis (Site) | 682.9 | ___ Diverticulosis | 562.10 | ___ Hepatitis | 573.3 | ___ Obesity | 278.0 |

DIAGNOSIS: (IF NOT CHECKED ABOVE)

SERVICES PERFORMED AT: ☐ Office ☐ E.R. ☐ ☐ ☐ CLAIM CONTAINS NO ORDERED REFERRING SERVICE

REFERRING PHYSICIAN & I.D. NUMBER

RETURN APPOINTMENT INFORMATION: 5 - 10 - 15 - 20 - 30 - 40 - 60 [ DAYS] [ WKS.] [ MOS.] [ PRN]

NEXT APPOINTMENT M - T - W - TH - F - S DATE / / TIME: AM PM

ACCEPT ASSIGNMENT? ☐ YES ☐ NO

DOCTOR'S SIGNATURE

**INSTRUCTIONS TO PATIENT FOR FILING INSURANCE CLAIMS:**

1. Complete upper portion of this form, sign and date.
2. Attach this form to your own insurance company's form for direct reimbursement.

**MEDICARE PATIENTS - DO NOT SEND THIS TO MEDICARE. WE WILL SUBMIT THE CLAIM FOR YOU.**

☐ CASH ☐ CHECK # ____ ☐ VISA ☐ MC ☐ CO-PAY

| TOTAL TODAY'S FEE | |
|---|---|
| OLD BALANCE | |
| TOTAL DUE | |
| AMOUNT REC'D. TODAY | |

INSUR-A-BILL ® BIBBERO SYSTEMS, INC. • PETALUMA, CA • UP. SUPER. © 6/94 (BIBB/STOCK)

Figure 10.5 Encounter Form

Source: Booth et al., *Medical Assisting,* 3e, p. 343. Copyright © 2005 The McGraw-Hill Companies, Inc. Reprinted with permission.

by the provider or the medical assistant. In other practices the patient may be handed the encounter form, which has been completed by the provider, and directed to the checkout area. The form will have billing information on it, as well as further instructions regarding future appointments and/or referrals to other practices.

Chapter 9 covered CPT and ICD-9 coding. The encounter form has that information on it for the checkout staff to enter into the practice management system. As discussed in Chapter 9, it is important to enter the primary diagnosis and to be certain that multiple procedure codes and diagnostic codes are linked properly.

Once the CPT and ICD-9 codes are entered into the system correctly, the copayment and coinsurance to be collected from the patient should be shown on the computer screen. However, not all management systems are accurately programmed, so the checkout staff may need to review the patient's insurance card to determine what the patient owes that day.

Depending on the practice, the encounter form may contain further instructions for the checkout staff. In a surgical or obstetrical practice, the patient will need to discuss payment options with a trained staff member, as most health plans do not cover the total cost of surgery or obstetrical care. A sample cost estimate form is shown in Figure 10.6. If your practice charges interest on unpaid balances, the patient must be provided information on the finance charges. Figure 10.7 illustrates a sample **federal truth-in-lending** form.



Date ________ Patient name ________ Date services to be provided ________

Procedure(s) ________________

The following is the estimated cost for the medical and or surgical services provided by Dr(s). ________. These costs do not include the charges from the anesthesiologist, pathologist, or the hospital or ambulatory surgery center.

Estimated cost ________ to ________

Estimated insurance payment ________ to ________

Patient balance ________ to ________

The above is an estimate only. The cost may vary if additional procedures/surgical services are necessary at the time of service. If a payment plan is necessary, please advise the counselor before the date of the medical/surgical services.

**Figure 10.6** Cost Estimate Form

Lending Statement
Federal Truth-in-Lending
Professional Services Provided

Patient name ______________
Address ________________________________________
Person responsible for account if patient is a minor or incompetent
______________________________
Address ________________________________________

1. Cash price for services $ _________
2. Cash down payment $ _________
3. Unpaid balance $ _________
4. Amount financed $ _________
5. Finance charge $ _________
6. Finance charge as annual percentage rate ______ %
7. Total amount of payment (line #4 plus line #5) $ _________
8. Deferred payment price (line #1 plus line #5) $ _________

Total payment due (#7 above) is payable to name of practice at the above address in monthly payments of $ _________. The first payment is payable on _________. Each subsequent payment is payable on the ______ day of each month until paid in full. The final payment is due on _________.

The patient has the right at any time to pay the unpaid balance due without penalty.

_______ ________________________________________
Date Patient signature or signature of responsible party

_______ ________________________________________
Date Physician or practice representative

**Figure 10.7** Truth-in-Lending form

## Processing an Established Patient

Established patients have already completed Steps 1 and 2 previously discussed. It is important, however, to check with patients at each visit to see if their information has changed. Patients sometimes find the question annoying, but often forget to tell their physician that they have moved or changed health care plans.

## Balancing the Day Sheet

Like all businesses, the medical practice must **balance** its books at the end of each day, as well as at the end of the month and the end of the financial year. For the daily close, this means that a member (or members) of the staff must ensure that all the appropriate charges have been entered for the day and that all the payments received from patients seen that day have been properly recorded on what is called a **day sheet** or **daily journal.** To do this in a computerized practice management system, follow these steps:

1. Get a copy of the day's appointment schedule from the check-in staff. Make sure they have indicated any cancellations or no-shows for the day.
2. Determine if you have an encounter form for every patient seen that day. This process should be done throughout the day to ensure that a patient doesn't accidentally leave the office with an encounter form. For any missing encounter forms, immediately contact the health care provider's medical assistant or nurse to determine why there is no form. The clinical staff can complete a new encounter form if the original form has been misplaced or if the patient accidentally took the form when leaving the office.
3. Once you have all encounter forms (or know why you will not have an encounter form for a particular patient), run a **trial balance/daily edit report.** The mechanics of requesting this report from your practice management system will differ depending on the software.
4. Verify that all activity listed on the encounter forms has been entered into the system. This simply means that every CPT and ICD-9 code has been entered for every patient seen that day.
5. Count the day's cash and then total the checks and credit card payments received for patients seen that day. Verify that the total amounts of cash, checks, and credit card payments match what the trial balance/daily edit report indicates for each type of payment.
6. If the day does not balance, an immediate review of each entry must be made. The usual errors are that a credit card entry was entered (posted) to cash, or a check was posted to cash, or something of that nature. Also, a payment amount may have been posted incorrectly (i.e., a $150 payment may have been entered as $15).
7. You must balance the day before you close the day if you are using a computerized system. Most practice management systems will not allow you to open a new day without the previous day being balanced. Also, most systems are programmed not to send the electronic claim forms on to the insurance companies and Medicare and Medicaid unless the day has balanced.

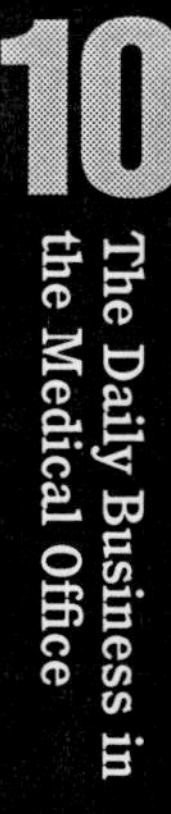

8. Medical practices submit their electronic billing to insurance companies and Medicare and Medicaid on a frequent basis, sometimes every day. The person responsible for this transmission varies from office to office. What is important to remember is that the information entered on a daily basis must be accurate to ensure timely payment of claims. The responsibility of entering patient data and services provided accurately is an important one.

A sample day sheet is found in Figure 10.8. This daily activity is part of the **bookkeeping** done in every practice. Bookkeeping involves both charges and payments, as we will see later on.



## Transmitting Claim Forms

The accepted claim form for outpatient services is called a **CMS-1500.** This form was developed by the federal government to ensure that information was provided to all payers in a similar fashion. Many insurance companies now allow or sometimes require electronic transmission of the CMS-1500. Medicare requires that all claims be electronically transmitted. For those insurance companies still accepting paper claims, the computerized PMS should generate the accepted CMS-1500 with the appropriate information completed. A staff member mails those claims to the required address. Whether the claims are electronically submitted or sent through the U.S. mail, it is important to get the claims to the payer quickly. A sample CMS-1500 is shown in Figure 10.9.

Some practices hire an outside billing company to handle all claim submittals and billing to patients. Because the information is entered electronically, this is sometimes a less expensive option than having staff process the claims. If using an outside company, it is important to clearly define its roles and responsibilities, and how much follow-up is expected. Whatever your practice chooses to do, the important thing to remember is that third-party payers can't pay claims they don't know exist!

## Processing the Payments

In today's electronic environment, many payments from insurance companies, Medicare, and Medicaid are electronically deposited to the practice's bank account. The practice receives a report, called a remittance voucher or remittance advice, that lists the individual payments on account for the patients. Depending on the practice's software, it is also possible to post the payment directly to the patient's account. Electronic posting is a valuable time saver, but it is important to verify the information as errors are possible. Additionally, payments will come from the patient after the date of service and need to be posted to the account appropriately. Any payment that comes after the date of service is called a "received on account" or ROA.

Family Care Center

**Patient Day Sheet**

9/4/2009 - 9/4/2009

| Entry | Date | Document | POS | Description | Provider | Code | Modifier | Amount |
|---|---|---|---|---|---|---|---|---|
| **BAREL000** | | **Ellen Barmenstein** | | | | | | |
| 222 | 9/4/2009 | 0909040000 | 11 | | 1 | 90658 | | 12.00 |
| 220 | 9/4/2009 | 0909040000 | 11 | | 1 | 99211 | | 30.00 |
| 221 | 9/4/2009 | 0909040000 | 11 | | 1 | 90471 | | 10.00 |
| | | Patient's Charges $52.00 | | Patient's Receipts $0.00 | Adjustments $0.00 | | Patient Balance $43.20 | |
| **BELSA001** | | **Sarina Bell** | | | | | | |
| 230 | 9/4/2009 | 0909040000 | 11 | | 1 | USLCOP | | -15.00 |
| 227 | 9/4/2009 | 0909040000 | 11 | | 1 | 99212 | | 44.00 |
| 228 | 9/4/2009 | 0909040000 | 11 | | 1 | 87430 | | 32.00 |
| 229 | 9/4/2009 | 0909040000 | 11 | | 1 | 85025 | 90 | 25.00 |
| | | Patient's Charges $101.00 | | Patient's Receipts -$15.00 | Adjustments $0.00 | | Patient Balance $86.00 | |
| **JONEL000** | | **Elizabeth Jones** | | | | | | |
| 226 | 9/4/2009 | 0909040000 | 11 | | 1 | USLCOP | | -15.00 |
| 225 | 9/4/2009 | 0909040000 | 11 | | 1 | 99212 | | 44.00 |
| | | Patient's Charges $44.00 | | Patient's Receipts -$15.00 | Adjustments $0.00 | | Patient Balance $88.00 | |
| **LOMCE000** | | **Cedera Lomos** | | | | | | |
| 214 | 9/4/2009 | 0909040000 | 11 | | 1 | 99204 | | 147.00 |
| | | Patient's Charges $147.00 | | Patient's Receipts $0.00 | Adjustments $0.00 | | Patient Balance $29.40 | |
| **LOMLI000** | | **Lisa Lomos** | | | | | | |
| 215 | 9/4/2009 | 0909040000 | 11 | | 1 | 99383 | | 140.00 |
| 216 | 9/4/2009 | 0909040000 | 11 | | 1 | 90465 | | 20.00 |
| 217 | 9/4/2009 | 0909040000 | 11 | | 1 | 90707 | | 105.00 |
| | | Patient's Charges $265.00 | | Patient's Receipts $0.00 | Adjustments $0.00 | | Patient Balance $53.00 | |
| **MITCA000** | | **Caroline Mitchell** | | | | | | |
| 231 | 9/4/2009 | 0909040000 | 11 | | 1 | 02 | | -60.00 |
| | | Patient's Charges $0.00 | | Patient's Receipts -$60.00 | Adjustments $0.00 | | Patient Balance $0.00 | |
| **PATLE000** | | **Leila Patterson** | | | | | | |
| 218 | 9/4/2009 | 0909040000 | 11 | | 1 | 99212 | | 44.00 |
| 219 | 9/4/2009 | 0909040000 | 11 | | 1 | 82465 | | 21.00 |
| | | Patient's Charges $65.00 | | Patient's Receipts $0.00 | Adjustments $0.00 | | Patient Balance $65.00 | |
| **TANHI000** | | **Hiro Tanaka** | | | | | | |
| 223 | 9/4/2009 | 0909040000 | 11 | | 1 | 99212 | | 44.00 |
| 224 | 9/4/2009 | 0909040000 | 11 | | 1 | TRICOP | | -10.00 |

**Figure 10.8** Day Sheet

Source: From Sanderson, *Patient Billing,* 6e. Copyright © 2008 The McGraw-Hill Companies, Inc. Reprinted with permission.

1500

**HEALTH INSURANCE CLAIM FORM**

APPROVED BY NATIONAL UNIFORM CLAIM COMMITTEE 08/05

PICA PICA

CARRIER

1. MEDICARE (Medicare #) MEDICAID (Medicaid #) TRICARE CHAMPUS (Sponsor's SSN) CHAMPVA (Member ID#) GROUP HEALTH PLAN (SSN or ID) FECA BLK LUNG (SSN) OTHER (ID)
1a. INSURED'S I.D. NUMBER (For Program in Item 1)
2. PATIENT'S NAME (Last Name, First Name, Middle Initial)
3. PATIENT'S BIRTH DATE MM DD YY SEX M F
4. INSURED'S NAME (Last Name, First Name, Middle Initial)
5. PATIENT'S ADDRESS (No., Street)
6. PATIENT RELATIONSHIP TO INSURED Self Spouse Child Other
7. INSURED'S ADDRESS (No., Street)
CITY STATE
8. PATIENT STATUS Single Married Other
CITY STATE
ZIP CODE TELEPHONE (Include Area Code) ( )
Employed Full-Time Student Part-Time Student
ZIP CODE TELEPHONE (Include Area Code) ( )
9. OTHER INSURED'S NAME (Last Name, First Name, Middle Initial)
10. IS PATIENT'S CONDITION RELATED TO:
11. INSURED'S POLICY GROUP OR FECA NUMBER
a. OTHER INSURED'S POLICY OR GROUP NUMBER
a. EMPLOYMENT? (Current or Previous) YES NO
a. INSURED'S DATE OF BIRTH MM DD YY SEX M F
b. OTHER INSURED'S DATE OF BIRTH MM DD YY SEX M F
b. AUTO ACCIDENT? YES NO PLACE (State)
b. EMPLOYER'S NAME OR SCHOOL NAME
c. EMPLOYER'S NAME OR SCHOOL NAME
c. OTHER ACCIDENT? YES NO
c. INSURANCE PLAN NAME OR PROGRAM NAME
d. INSURANCE PLAN NAME OR PROGRAM NAME
10d. RESERVED FOR LOCAL USE
d. IS THERE ANOTHER HEALTH BENEFIT PLAN? YES NO *If yes*, return to and complete item 9 a-d.

READ BACK OF FORM BEFORE COMPLETING & SIGNING THIS FORM.

12. PATIENT'S OR AUTHORIZED PERSON'S SIGNATURE I authorize the release of any medical or other information necessary to process this claim. I also request payment of government benefits either to myself or to the party who accepts assignment below.

SIGNED DATE

13. INSURED'S OR AUTHORIZED PERSON'S SIGNATURE I authorize payment of medical benefits to the undersigned physician or supplier for services described below.

SIGNED

PATIENT AND INSURED INFORMATION

14. DATE OF CURRENT: MM DD YY ILLNESS (First symptom) OR INJURY (Accident) OR PREGNANCY(LMP)
15. IF PATIENT HAS HAD SAME OR SIMILAR ILLNESS. GIVE FIRST DATE MM DD YY
16. DATES PATIENT UNABLE TO WORK IN CURRENT OCCUPATION MM DD YY FROM TO MM DD YY
17. NAME OF REFERRING PROVIDER OR OTHER SOURCE
17a.
17b. NPI
18. HOSPITALIZATION DATES RELATED TO CURRENT SERVICES MM DD YY FROM TO MM DD YY
19. RESERVED FOR LOCAL USE
20. OUTSIDE LAB? YES NO $ CHARGES
21. DIAGNOSIS OR NATURE OF ILLNESS OR INJURY (Relate Items 1, 2, 3 or 4 to Item 24E by Line)
1.
2.
3.
4.
22. MEDICAID RESUBMISSION CODE ORIGINAL REF. NO.
23. PRIOR AUTHORIZATION NUMBER

| 24. A. DATE(S) OF SERVICE From MM DD YY To MM DD YY | B. PLACE OF SERVICE | C. EMG | D. PROCEDURES, SERVICES, OR SUPPLIES (Explain Unusual Circumstances) CPT/HCPCS MODIFIER | E. DIAGNOSIS POINTER | F. $ CHARGES | G. DAYS OR UNITS | H. EPSDT Family Plan | I. ID. QUAL. | J. RENDERING PROVIDER ID. # |
|---|---|---|---|---|---|---|---|---|---|
| 1 | | | | | | | | NPI | |
| 2 | | | | | | | | NPI | |
| 3 | | | | | | | | NPI | |
| 4 | | | | | | | | NPI | |
| 5 | | | | | | | | NPI | |
| 6 | | | | | | | | NPI | |

25. FEDERAL TAX I.D. NUMBER SSN EIN
26. PATIENT'S ACCOUNT NO.
27. ACCEPT ASSIGNMENT? (For govt. claims, see back) YES NO
28. TOTAL CHARGE $
29. AMOUNT PAID $
30. BALANCE DUE $
31. SIGNATURE OF PHYSICIAN OR SUPPLIER INCLUDING DEGREES OR CREDENTIALS (I certify that the statements on the reverse apply to this bill and are made a part thereof.)
SIGNED DATE
32. SERVICE FACILITY LOCATION INFORMATION
a. NPI b.
33. BILLING PROVIDER INFO & PH # ( )
a. NPI b.

PHYSICIAN OR SUPPLIER INFORMATION

NUCC Instruction Manual available at: www.nucc.org *PLEASE PRINT OR TYPE* APPROVED OMB-0938-0999 FORM CMS-1500 (08-05)

SAMPLE

**Figure 10.9** CMS-1500 (continued)

Source: www.cms.hhs.gov/cmsforms/downloads/CMS1500805.pdf.

BECAUSE THIS FORM IS USED BY VARIOUS GOVERNMENT AND PRIVATE HEALTH PROGRAMS, SEE SEPARATE INSTRUCTIONS ISSUED BY APPLICABLE PROGRAMS.

NOTICE: Any person who knowingly files a statement of claim containing any misrepresentation or any false, incomplete or misleading information may be guilty of a criminal act punishable under law and may be subject to civil penalties.

REFERS TO GOVERNMENT PROGRAMS ONLY

MEDICARE AND CHAMPUS PAYMENTS. A patient's signature requests that payment be made and authorizes release of any information necessary to process the claim and certifies that the information provided in Blocks 1 through 12 is true, accurate and complete. In the case of a Medicare claim, the patient's signature authorizes any entity to release to Medicare medical and nonmedical information, including employment status, and whether the person has employer group health insurance, liability, no fault, worker's compensation or other insurance which is responsible to pay for the services for which the Medicare claim is made. See 42 CFR 411.24(a). If item 9 is completed, the patient's signature authorizes release of the information to the health plan or agency shown. In Medicare assigned or CHAMPUS participation cases, the physician agrees to accept the charge determination of the Medicare carrier or CHAMPUS fiscal intermediary as the full charge, and the patient is responsible only for the deductible, coinsurance and noncovered services. Coinsurance and the deductible are based upon the charge determination of the Medicare carrier or CHAMPUS fiscal intermediary if this is less than the charge submitted. CHAMPUS is not a health insurance program but makes payment for health benefits provided through certain affiliations with the Uniformed Services. Information on the patient's sponsor should be provided in those items captioned in "Insured"; i.e., items 1a, 4, 6, 7, 9, and 11.

BLACK LUNG AND FECA CLAIMS

The provider agrees to accept the amount paid by the Government as payment in full. See Black Lung and FECA instructions regarding required procedure and diagnosis coding systems.

SIGNATURE OF PHYSICIAN OR SUPPLIER (MEDICARE, CHAMPUS, FECA AND BLACK LUNG)

I certify that the services shown on this form were medically indicated and necessary for the health of the patient and were personally furnished by me or were furnished incident to my professional service by my employee under my immediate personal supervision, except as otherwise expressly permitted by Medicare or CHAMPUS regulations.

For services to be considered as "incident" to a physician's professional service, 1) they must be rendered under the physician's immediate personal supervision by his/her employee, 2) they must be an integral, although incidental part of a covered physician's service, 3) they must be of kinds commonly furnished in physician's offices, and 4) the services of nonphysicians must be included on the physician's bills.

For CHAMPUS claims, I further certify that I (or any employee) who rendered services am not an active duty member of the Uniformed Services or a civilian employee of the United States Government or a contract employee of the United States Government, either civilian or military (refer to 5 USC 5536). For Black-Lung claims, I further certify that the services performed were for a Black Lung-related disorder.

No Part B Medicare benefits may be paid unless this form is received as required by existing law and regulations (42 CFR 424.32).

NOTICE: Any one who misrepresents or falsifies essential information to receive payment from Federal funds requested by this form may upon conviction be subject to fine and imprisonment under applicable Federal laws.

NOTICE TO PATIENT ABOUT THE COLLECTION AND USE OF MEDICARE, CHAMPUS, FECA, AND BLACK LUNG INFORMATION (PRIVACY ACT STATEMENT)

We are authorized by CMS, CHAMPUS and OWCP to ask you for information needed in the administration of the Medicare, CHAMPUS, FECA, and Black Lung programs. Authority to collect information is in section 205(a), 1862, 1872 and 1874 of the Social Security Act as amended, 42 CFR 411.24(a) and 424.5(a) (6), and 44 USC 3101;41 CFR 101 et seq and 10 USC 1079 and 1086; 5 USC 8101 et seq; and 30 USC 901 et seq; 38 USC 613; E.O. 9397.

The information we obtain to complete claims under these programs is used to identify you and to determine your eligibility. It is also used to decide if the services and supplies you received are covered by these programs and to insure that proper payment is made.

The information may also be given to other providers of services, carriers, intermediaries, medical review boards, health plans, and other organizations or Federal agencies, for the effective administration of Federal provisions that require other third parties payers to pay primary to Federal program, and as otherwise necessary to administer these programs. For example, it may be necessary to disclose information about the benefits you have used to a hospital or doctor. Additional disclosures are made through routine uses for information contained in systems of records.

**FOR MEDICARE CLAIMS:** See the notice modifying system No. 09-70-0501, titled, 'Carrier Medicare Claims Record,' published in the Federal Register, Vol. 55 No. 177, page 37549, Wed. Sept. 12, 1990, or as updated and republished.

**FOR OWCP CLAIMS:** Department of Labor, Privacy Act of 1974, "Republication of Notice of Systems of Records," Federal Register Vol. 55 No. 40, Wed Feb. 28, 1990, See ESA-5, ESA-6, ESA-12, ESA-13, ESA-30, or as updated and republished.

**FOR CHAMPUS CLAIMS:** PRINCIPLE PURPOSE(S): To evaluate eligibility for medical care provided by civilian sources and to issue payment upon establishment of eligibility and determination that the services/supplies received are authorized by law.

ROUTINE USE(S): Information from claims and related documents may be given to the Dept. of Veterans Affairs, the Dept. of Health and Human Services and/or the Dept. of Transportation consistent with their statutory administrative responsibilities under CHAMPUS/CHAMPVA; to the Dept. of Justice for representation of the Secretary of Defense in civil actions; to the Internal Revenue Service, private collection agencies, and consumer reporting agencies in connection with recoupment claims; and to Congressional Offices in response to inquiries made at the request of the person to whom a record pertains. Appropriate disclosures may be made to other federal, state, local, foreign government agencies, private business entities, and individual providers of care, on matters relating to entitlement, claims adjudication, fraud, program abuse, utilization review, quality assurance, peer review, program integrity, third-party liability, coordination of benefits, and civil and criminal litigation related to the operation of CHAMPUS.

DISCLOSURES: Voluntary; however, failure to provide information will result in delay in payment or may result in denial of claim. With the one exception discussed below, there are no penalties under these programs for refusing to supply information. However, failure to furnish information regarding the medical services rendered or the amount charged would prevent payment of claims under these programs. Failure to furnish any other information, such as name or claim number, would delay payment of the claim. Failure to provide medical information under FECA could be deemed an obstruction.

It is mandatory that you tell us if you know that another party is responsible for paying for your treatment. Section 1128B of the Social Security Act and 31 USC 3801-3812 provide penalties for withholding this information.

You should be aware that P.L. 100-503, the "Computer Matching and Privacy Protection Act of 1988", permits the government to verify information by way of computer matches.

MEDICAID PAYMENTS (PROVIDER CERTIFICATION)

I hereby agree to keep such records as are necessary to disclose fully the extent of services provided to individuals under the State's Title XIX plan and to furnish information regarding any payments claimed for providing such services as the State Agency or Dept. of Health and Human Services may request.

I further agree to accept, as payment in full, the amount paid by the Medicaid program for those claims submitted for payment under that program, with the exception of authorized deductible, coinsurance, co-payment or similar cost-sharing charge.

**SIGNATURE OF PHYSICIAN (OR SUPPLIER):** I certify that the services listed above were medically indicated and necessary to the health of this patient and were personally furnished by me or my employee under my personal direction.

NOTICE: This is to certify that the foregoing information is true, accurate and complete. I understand that payment and satisfaction of this claim will be from Federal and State funds, and that any false claims, statements, or documents, or concealment of a material fact, may be prosecuted under applicable Federal or State laws.

According to the Paperwork Reduction Act of 1995, no persons are required to respond to a collection of information unless it displays a valid OMB control number. The valid OMB control number for this information collection is 0938-0999. The time required to complete this information collection is estimated to average 10 minutes per response, including the time to review instructions, search existing data resources, gather the data needed, and complete and review the information collection. If you have any comments concerning the accuracy of the time estimate(s) or suggestions for improving this form, please write to: CMS, Attn: PRA Reports Clearance Officer, 7500 Security Boulevard, Baltimore, Maryland 21244-1850. This address is for comments and/or suggestions only. DO NOT MAIL COMPLETED CLAIM FORMS TO THIS ADDRESS.



**Figure 10.9** (concluded)

## Managing the Accounts Receivable

**Accounts receivable** is the money owed to the practice—either from the patient directly or from an insurance company, Medicare, Medicaid, or other third-party payer. The longer someone owes money, the less likely it is that the bill will be paid, so it is important to manage the accounts receivable (AR) on a frequent basis.

Many practices have a staff member in the business office whose responsibilities are to work the AR. In large practices, there may be someone working the Medicare accounts, someone else working the insurance companies, and a third person working the cash balances. Working the accounts means to follow up on payment.



The practice management system can provide a variety of reports to aid in collecting the AR. Reports can be produced that provide balances by payer type (Medicare, Medicaid, Blue Cross, Aetna, etc.) as well as reports that reflect the age of the balance, usually in 30-, 60-, 90-, and 120-day increments. The age of the balance means how long the money has been due to the practice. Remember, the longer the money has been owed, the less likely it is that you will get payment, so a good AR will have small amounts in its 60-day or more column.

To work the insurance accounts receivable, it is important to review the reports, called remittance vouchers or advices, that come to the practice either electronically or through the U.S. mail. These reports should be reviewed as soon as they are received, for they contain valuable information about the status of claims. If a claim is being denied for payment by an insurance company or Medicare/Medicaid, the remittance voucher will tell the reader why the claim is being denied.

Claims are often denied for a variety of reasons. Three common reasons a claim has been denied include:

- The patient has not met the deductible.
- The patient is no longer insured by the insurance company.
- The type of services provided are not covered by the insurance company.

If the claim is denied for any of these reasons, the balanced owed is the responsibility of the patient. The business office makes an entry into the patient's account, moving the balance owed from an insurance balance to a patient pay balance (or cash balance). It is important to immediately send a bill to the patient, to make the patient aware that the bill is his or her responsibility.

Claims may also be denied because the practice has made an error in submitting the claim. Here are some common errors:

- Wrong policy or group number.
- Wrong date of birth.

- Procedure code and diagnostic code are not properly linked.
- Provider not listed.
- Other required information is not listed.

When the claim is denied because the practice made an error in submitting the claim, it is important to correct the error and resubmit the claim right away. Many insurance companies have a short time span available for consideration of resubmitted claims.

Some insurance companies now provide electronic access for providers to view the status of the claim. Because of the secure nature of those websites, practices must have signed up for the services and have appropriate passwords.

Working the cash receivables is a different process for the business office staff. To make their jobs easier and to comply with the third-party payer requirements, collecting copays at time of service is critical. Failure to do so could result in the loss of participating status with some third-party payers. Also, it just makes sense to get as much of the payment up front as possible. Some practices ask patients to pay the copay before they see their health care provider.

Assuming that the front office (both check-in and checkout) staff are doing a good job collecting copays, the cash balances usually represent the coinsurance or deductible. The cash balances on a patient's account also represent those services that the patient's insurance company did not cover.

In Chapter 8, the concept of charges versus payments was covered. Here is another way to look at this confusing concept.

If you purchase a pair of jeans at your local department store, there is a set price for those jeans. Even if they are on sale, there is still a set price. The department store sets the price. You, as the payer, can either buy the jeans or not buy the jeans. For health care charges, the provider sets the price for each service, just like the department store sets the price for the jeans. The difference is that the patient is not usually the payer of services (the jeans); the insurance company is the payer. Also, the patient is not usually choosing the services (the jeans); the provider is determining the services and you *need* the services, not *want* services. The patient may *want* the jeans, but the patient does not *need* the jeans, something parents having been saying to their children for many, many years!

In this country, the third-party payers determine what the payment will be for the service. Why don't providers just set their price at what the third-party payers will pay? For a very simple reason: Every third-party payer has a different payment for each service.

For the business office staff collecting cash balances, a more personal touch is often necessary. First, if the cash balance is a result of nonpayment by a third-party

Name of Practice

Date ________ Patient name __________

The following is the balance owed for the medical and or surgical services provided by Dr(s). __________. This balance will be paid in ______ equal payments of __________. Payments will be due on the __________ day of each month.

Failure to maintain this payment plan could result in the patient's account being sent to a collection agency.

______________ ________________________________

Date Patient or Responsible Party

**Figure 10.10** Payment Plan



payer, the patient is often confused and angry. It is important to clearly explain to the patient why the third-party payer is not paying, and why the balance is the patient's responsibility.

Second, depending on the size of the balance, it may be necessary to set up a payment plan for the patient. As with patients having elective services, it is important to set up a plan in writing and to monitor the patient's payments. A sample payment plan is shown in Figure 10.10. If it is the practice's policy to charge interest on unpaid balances, a federal truth-in-lending form (Figure 10.7) must also be completed. When establishing a payment plan, it is important to have the balance paid off in the shortest amount of time possible. For example, if a patient owes a balance of $1,000, the monthly payments should be at least $100. Although small monthly payments may seem like a good thing to do for our patients, it creates more problems than it will solve.

Patients do not pay their bills for a variety of reasons and collecting cash balances is difficult. A system needs to be in place to monitor payments. Although phone calls are certainly appropriate when a patient has not made payments, the likelihood is that you will need a good set of collection letters to use. It is important to monitor cash balances, because the longer the money is owed, the less likely it is to be collected. Figures 10.11, 10.12, and 10.13 illustrate a series of letters that may be used.

Finally, health care practices must also make the difficult decision to send a patient's account to a collection agency. Many practices do not do this, preferring to **write off** the balance to bad debt. If the choice is made to send the patient's account to

Name of Practice
Address
(use letterhead)

Date

Patient Name
Address
City, State Zip

Dear Mr./Mrs. Last Name of Patient

In our busy lives, we sometimes forget to make payments on our accounts with our doctors. We know that you may have just overlooked this payment, but your account with our practice is now overdue.

Please submit a payment of $ ________ within the next 10 days.

Do not hesitate to contact me if you have any questions or concerns.

Sincerely,

Name of Staff Person
Patient Account Coordinator

**Figure 10.11** Collection Letter Number One

Name of Practice
Address
(use letterhead)
(Send 20 days after letter #1)

Date

Patient Name
Address
City, State Zip

Dear Mr./Mrs. Last Name of Patient

We still haven't received payment from you on your account with our practice. Failure to resolve this matter within the next 10 days could result in your account being forwarded to a collection agency for action. We do not wish to take this step, so please make arrangements to take care of this balance immediately.

**Figure 10.12** Collection Letter Number Two (continued)

*(concluded)*

Please submit a payment of $ ______ within the next 5 days.

Please call me within the next 3 business days at XXX-XXX-XXXX so that we may finalize a resolution to this overdue balance.

Your attention to this matter is greatly appreciated.

Sincerely,

Name of Staff Person
Patient Account Coordinator

**Figure 10.12** (concluded)



Name of Practice
Address
(use letterhead)
(Send 10 days after letter #2)

Date

Patient Name
Address
City, State Zip

Dear Mr./Mrs. Last Name of Patient

Your account with us is now seriously delinquent. We have sent you two requests for payment and have not heard from you.

If a payment of $ ________ is not made within the next 10 days, your account will be turned over to a collection agency for action. It is also possible that Dr. ________ will determine that you should be dismissed from our practice.

Your immediate attention to this past due balance is important. Payment is due no later than ________ (date).

Sincerely,

Name of Staff Person
Patient Account Coordinator

cc: Dr. __________

**Figure 10.13** Collection Letter Number Three

Name of Practice
Address
(use letterhead)

Date
(Send certified mail, but also send in regular mail)

Patient Name
Address
City, State Zip

Dear Mr./Mrs. Last Name of Patient

It is with deep regret that I must inform you that I am withdrawing from further medical care for you due to your nonpayment of your account (or whatever other reason, such as noncompliance with recommended care).

You will need to find another physician to take over in your medical care. I will be available to attend to you for the next thirty (30 days) until ________ (date). That will give you time to find another physician.

A request for release of information is enclosed. Please complete this form and return it to our office so that we may forward your medical records to your new physician.

Very truly yours,

Name of Physician, MD or DO

enc.

**Figure 10.14** Dismissal from Practice Letter

collections, it is important to let the patient know that you are going to take that step (see Figure 10.13).

When a patient's balance is sent to a collection agency, the practice management system should reflect a zero balance. Good systems flag the patient's account so that before the patient is seen again, payment is made.

Once the account is sent to collections, many practices dismiss the patient from the practice. This letter informs the patient that the provider is no longer willing to care for him or her. A sample letter is illustrated in Figure 10.14. This letter should always be signed by the provider to ensure that there is no continuity of care issue with the patient. Some states have very specific language that must be used in a dismissal letter, so check with your local medical society to make sure you use the appropriate language.

## Summary

Unlike most businesses where simple financial transactions take place, physician practices must meet a complicated set of requirements to collect payment. It is critical that all staff members have a basic understanding of the financial operation of the practice. Attention to detail on a daily basis by staff and providers alike is vital to the success of the practice and will help make it profitable. Everyone in the practice should be able to respond to basic questions about the payment process.

# Office Safety and Wellness

# Part 4

## Office Safety and Wellness

# Chapter 11

# Safety in the Medical Office

## Introduction

*The health and safety of the physicians, staff, patients, and other visitors should always be a top priority in the medical office. Providing a physically safe environment not only makes common sense, but it also makes good business sense. All practices should have appropriate measures in place to protect the patients and staff.*

*In this chapter we will review the federal requirements for health and safety in the workplace. We will look at some of the infection control issues all offices face. Last, we will discuss what to do in the event a pandemic strikes your community. Chapter 12 addresses the safety of the records in the office.*

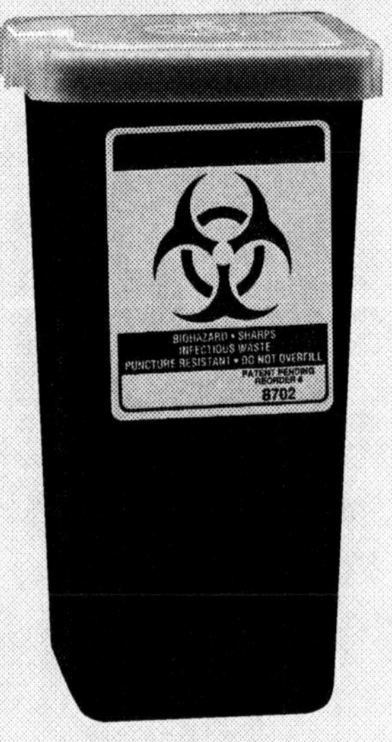


## Chapter Outline

# OSHA Compliance Program

The **Occupational Safety and Health Administration (OSHA)** is the federal agency that works to prevent injuries and protect the health of the American workplace. OSHA is part of the U.S. Department of Labor, but OSHA staff work closely with the individual states in establishing guidelines and standards to promote worker safety and health. There are general guidelines issued by OSHA, and your state may have additional guidelines in the area of office safety as well. All employers, regardless of the size of the organization, are required to follow OSHA standards. Although OSHA does not currently require medical and dental offices to maintain an official log of reportable injuries and illnesses using OSHA Form 300, you may be required to do so under state laws.

There are six OSHA standards that apply to all medical offices and a seventh standard that applies if you offer X-ray services in your office.

The first standard is the *bloodborne pathogens* standard. Congress updated the rule when it passed the Needlestick Safety and Prevention Act in 2000. The intent of this standard is to reduce exposure to bloodborne diseases. The rule specifically targets the human immunodeficiency virus (HIV) and the hepatitis B and C viruses. The basic rules require the following:

- A written exposure control plan, updated annually. The update should reflect any changes in technology (the use of newer, safer devices in order to reduce risk of needlesticks, for example). The plan doesn't require the use of every new device on the market, only documentation as to why you chose the specific devices. The plan should also document input from employees when selecting various devices.
- Use of safer needles and sharps.
- Use of the right personal protective equipment (PPE). This includes gloves, face and eye protection, and gowns.
- Use of universal precautions.
- No-cost hepatitis B vaccinations for staff who may have exposure.
- Medical follow-up after an exposure incident.
- Proper containment of all regulated waste.
- Identification (via labels or color-coding) of regulated waste containers, sharps disposal boxes, and containers for disposal of hazardous waste.
- Employee training.

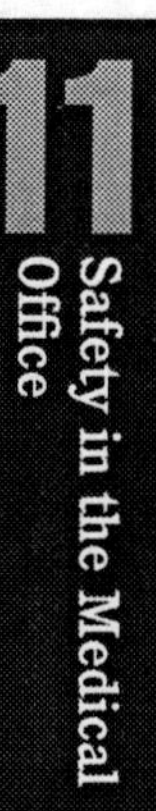

The second OSHA standard is the *hazard communication* standard. Under this standard, if your office contains any hazardous chemicals of any kind, the employees have a right to know about them. Every medical office contains some hazardous chemicals. Alcohol, disinfectants, anesthetic agents, and sterilizing agents are examples. The safety officer should have collected the manufacturer-supplied Material Safety Data Sheets (MSDS) that outline the proper procedures for working with a specific substance, as well as how to contain the material in the event of a spill or other emergency. If an MSDS has been misplaced, a simple Internet search will provide the safety officer with a variety of resources to get a new MSDS. Just enter "MSDS" into any search engine. It is a good idea to keep the sheets in separate sheet protectors, and to clearly label the notebook.

Having *clearly marked exit routes* is the third standard under OSHA. All offices must provide safe and accessible building exits in case of fire or other emergencies. Accessible means they cannot be blocked or locked from the inside. At a very minimum, you must establish exit routes to accommodate all employees and patients in a defined workspace. The easiest way to remember what to do in the case of fire or other emergency that requires everyone to evacuate is to remember the acronym RACE. Figure 11.1 outlines RACE. Every office should have a fire drill at least once a year, preferably twice a year.



OSHA's fourth standard deals with the *safe use and location of electrical outlets and wiring in hazardous locations.* If you use flammable gases, you may need special wiring and equipment installation. In these cases, it is important to check with your local fire department or to ask for an OSHA consult.

Currently, medical and dental offices are exempt under federal law from the fifth standard. This standard requires the *reporting of occupational injuries and illnesses.* However, your state law may be different. You can go to the OSHA website and search for states

*R*—remove all patients or visitors that are in immediate danger.
*A*—activate the fire alarm and call 911. Notify the supervisor or administrator in charge.
*C*—close all doors and windows to prevent the fire from spreading. Be certain all exam and diagnostic areas are empty before closing the doors.
*E*—extinguish the fire if possible. Do this only if is safe to do so.

**Figure 11.1** Fire Procedures

with OSHA-approved health and safety programs to see if your state has a separate set of procedures.

The final OSHA guideline for all offices is the requirement to *display the notice of employee rights in a conspicuous place in the office.* Usually these posters are found in the employee break room. The posters may be downloaded from OSHA's website (see Figure 11.2) or ordered free of charge by calling OSHA.

The seventh OSHA standard applies to *X-ray machines or other imaging services.* This standard requires:

- A survey of the types of radiation used in the facility, including X-rays.
- Restricted areas to limit employee exposures.
- Employees working in restricted areas to wear personal radiation monitors such as film badges or pocket dosimeters.
- Rooms and equipment to be labeled and equipped with caution signs.

OSHA offers a variety of website resources, as shown in Figure 11.2. It is also important to check with your state's health and safety department to see if you are subject to additional rules.

OSHA requires that one employee be designated as a safety officer. This person is responsible for developing and maintaining the OSHA safety programs. The safety officer creates and updates the safety manual and trains all new employees in the safety standards. Employees must annually review OSHA safety programs, and the safety officer must also annually review the rules to ensure that they are up-to-date. In addition, the safety officer is responsible for all recordkeeping requirements imposed by OSHA or the state health and safety office, as well as representing the facility in the event of an inspection by OSHA or the state.

OSHA has a general duty clause in its regulations. This means that either the safety officer, practice administrator, or physician administrator must review the facility's physical space for adequate lighting, appropriate signage for exiting, safe stairs and stairways, and air quality. Additionally, an evaluation of the fire safety system in place as well as evacuation procedures is important. If automated external defibrillators are in place, the safety officer is responsible for their proper installation and the training of appropriate personnel.

Generally, OSHA investigations occur in response to written, signed complaints. The majority of these complaints are handled by phone and fax. OSHA first does an informal alert to the medical office with a warning that the office may not be in compliance. OSHA will ask the office to address the problem and inform OSHA of the actions taken to correct

*Bloodborne pathogens and hazard communications*—This publication combines the two important OSHA standards regarding bloodborne pathogens and hazardous materials communication. It is available in a PDF file or an html file. Go to www.osha.gov and search Publications. The current publication number is 3186-06N.

*OSHA notice of employee rights*—This notice is required to be posted in all offices and workplaces. A sample notice is available in both English and Spanish at www.osha.gov (search Publications). The current publication number is 3165. It is available as a PDF file.

*Needlestick safety programs*—There are several different resources from the National Institute for Safety and Health (NIOSH) and the Centers for Disease Control and Prevention (CDC). A workbook for designing, implementing, and evaluating a sharps injury prevention program is available at www.cdc.gov by searching for the keywords "sharps safety." Additionally, on the NIOSH website (www.cdc.gov/niosh) you can search for more information about safer medical device implementation in health care facilities. NIOSH is the federal agency responsible for conducting research and making recommendations for the prevention of work-related injury and illness. NIOSH is part of the CDC in the U.S. Department of Health and Human Services.

*Personal protective equipment*—An overview of regulations regarding personal protective equipment is available at the OSHA website. It is available in a PDF file or an html file. Go to www.osha.gov and search Publications. The current publication number is 3151.

*Small business handbook*—This is a great overview of all the OSHA requirements for small business. Go to www.osha.gov and search Publications using the keywords "small business." It is available as a PDF or an html file.

*Evacuation plan*—This site has great checklists and procedures for developing your evacuation plan. Go to www.osha.gov and search using the keywords "evacuation plans and procedures." There are printable checklists and ideas for training available on the site.

**Figure 11.2** OSHA Website Resources



the deficiency. However, if it is a serious violation, or the office has a history of citations, OSHA will do an on-site inspection. Although these inspections are normally limited to the area where the violation occurred, an inspector may document other violations that are in plain sight. The inspectors may also ask to see your written exposure control plan and other logs and related records. Citations carry a specific monetary policy. Medical practices will have a fixed amount of time to correct the problem. Additionally, your state or local health department may have the legal right to inspect your office at any time.

Knowing and following the state and local laws regarding health and safety are important for everyone involved.

## Preventing the Transfer of Disease in the Office

As mentioned, OSHA requires that all offices have an infection control plan in place. **Infection control** is the effort made, often regulated by the federal or state government, to control the presence of harmful microorganisms. Everyone in the office is responsible for maintaining a safe working environment. Much of the work to ensure this safe working environment is the responsibility of the clinical staff; however, all staff should have an understanding of how disease is spread.

We have all used the words *bugs* or *germs* to describe an illness we have had that we believe we caught from someone or something else. These bugs and germs are microbes that cause disease. The microbes are called pathogens, and most pathogens belong to one of four groups—viruses, fungi, bacteria, and protozoa.

Viruses are tiny bits of protein-coated nucleic acid that take over cells in another living organism. Viruses need living cells to reproduce. The flu and the common cold are viruses.

Fungi are plantlike organisms. They live in the air, the soil, on other plants, and in water. Mushrooms and mold are the most commonly known fungi. Only some fungi cause disease. There is evidence that our bodies may react adversely to mold. Ringworm is another example of a disease caused by a fungus.

Bacteria are one-celled creatures found in water and soil, and also on other organisms. There are thousands of different types of bacteria in the world and many are harmless. Some are even helpful to humans. However, some bacteria cause disease. The most commonly known problem caused by bacteria is strep throat. This problem is caused by a bacteria called *streptococcus A.* Bacteria may also form spores. A spore is a protective protein shield that bacteria form around themselves. The bacteria rest until the right conditions exist for growing.

Protozoa are tiny parasites that live in or on another organism. Found mostly in tropical or moist environments, they can cause diseases like malaria.

Most pathogens live in our environment, but they don't always cause disease. The chain of infection has five links, as illustrated in Figure 11.3.

The process of infection is like a chain with five links. The first link is the **reservoir host,** the animal, human, or insect where the microorganism lives and grows. Sometimes the reservoir host shows signs of infection, but sometimes it does not. The reservoir host is the carrier of the microorganism.

The second link is the exit from the reservoir. Some of the exit routes include the nose or mouth, the urinary tract, the intestinal tract, or a wound.

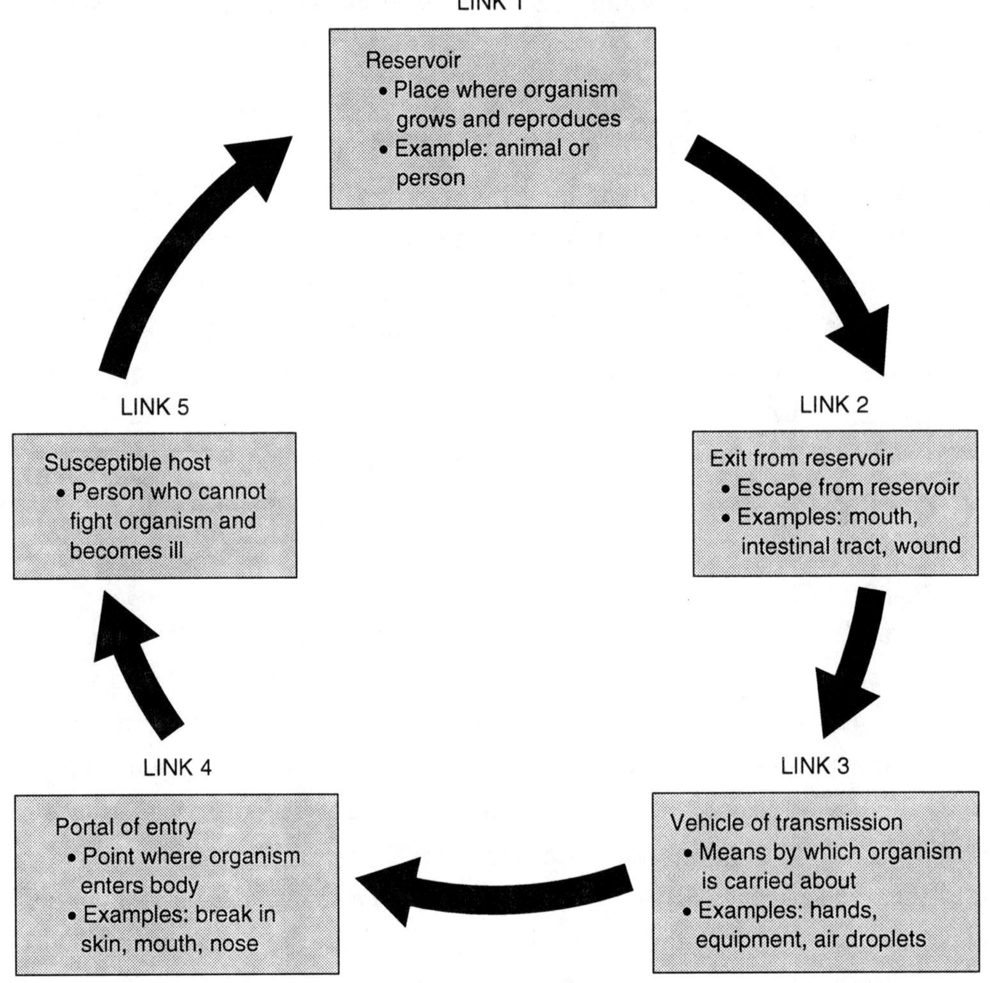


**Figure 11.3** Process of Infection



The third link in the process is called the vehicle of transmission. This is the way the organisms are carried about. Hands, equipment, instruments, silverware and linens, and air droplets are examples of vehicles of transmission.

A portal of entry is the fourth link in the cycle. The pathogen must have nutrients to survive, so the portal of entry is where the microorganism can enter the next host's body. The microbes may be in air droplets that we breathe. Some microbes may be found in food or drink. An open cut can be a portal of entry.

The final link is a susceptible host. This is a person who cannot fight the pathogen once it has entered the body. He or she becomes ill. The new host also becomes a carrier, or reservoir host, and the infection chain may start again.

Some pathogens make you sick for a short time, some for a long time. There are three types of infection—acute, chronic, or latent.

An acute infection develops quickly and lasts for a short time. The flu is an example. The immune system works to destroy the virus and the symptoms disappear in one to two weeks.

A chronic infection lasts for a long time—sometimes for a lifetime. Symptoms may not always be present. Hepatitis B is an example of a chronic infection caused by a virus. The virus may be detectable only in the patient's bloodstream, and the patient may have no symptoms.

When a pathogen has not been active (dormant), it is called a latent infection. Viruses can cause these kinds of infections. Genital herpes is an example of a dormant infection. When the pathogen becomes active, the virus may be transmitted to other people. Table 11.1 illustrates some common infectious diseases and how they are spread.

There are two types of transmission of infectious diseases. Direct transmission is when there is direct contact between the reservoir host and the susceptible host. Direct transmission includes:

- Touching blood or other infected body fluids of the reservoir host
- Inhaling infected air droplets of the reservoir host
- Intimate contact such as kissing or sexual intercourse
- Shaking hands

**Table 11.1** Common Infectious Diseases

| Infectious Disease | How It Is Spread |
|---|---|
| Chicken pox | Direct contact or droplets |
| *E. coli* bacteria | Contaminated food |
| Giardiasis | Direct contact with infected fecal matter or water containing feces |
| Hepatitis B | Direct contact with infectious body fluid |
| HIV/AIDS | Direct contact with infectious body fluid |
| Influenza (flu) | Droplets in the air, direct contact with infected carriers or contaminated articles |
| Measles | Infected droplets |
| Mononucleosis | Infected droplets |
| Pneumonia | Infected droplets |
| Rabies | Direct contact with saliva of infected animal usually through an animal bite |
| Viral meningitis | Direct contact with respiratory secretions such as saliva or sputum |

Indirect transmission is when the pathogens are spread through a vector. **Vectors** are objects that contain pathogens. Some examples of vectors are:

- Using a medical instrument that has not been properly disinfected
- Getting bitten by an insect that carries the disease
- Eating food that is contaminated
- Drinking from an infected person's glass
- Touching a contaminated surface, such as doorknob or a child's toy

In the office, it is necessary to break this chain so that the microorganism is no longer able to live. The methods and practices designed to prevent the spread of disease are referred to as **medical asepsis.**

The most important medical aseptic practice is washing your hands. Learning the correct way to wash your hands is important. Figure 11.4 outlines the proper hand-washing technique.

When should you wash your hands? Before and after patient contact or contact with blood or other bodily fluids; after coughing, sneezing, or blowing your nose; before and after lunch; after using the restroom; and after any contact with contaminated material. Clinical personnel routinely wear latex gloves when handling anything that could pose a risk of contamination.



There is much evidence to suggest that proper hand-washing, as well as covering your mouth when coughing or sneezing, goes a long way in preventing infection. Figure 11.5

1. Remove all jewelry. A plain wedding band may be left on and scrubbed.
2. Turn on faucets using a paper towel, and adjust water temperature to moderately warm.
3. Wet your hands and apply liquid soap.
4. Work the soap into a lather, making sure that both hands are lathered. Rub vigorously for two minutes. Keep hands lower than your forearms so that dirty water flows into the sink instead of back on your arms. Interlace your fingers to clean between them, and keep your fingertips pointed down.
5. Use a nailbrush or orange stick to clean under your nails and cuticles.
6. Rinse your hands well, keeping your hands lower than your forearms.
7. With the water still running, dry your hands thoroughly with clean dry paper towels. Turn off the faucet using a clean dry paper towel. Discard the towel.

**Figure 11.4** Aseptic Hand-Washing

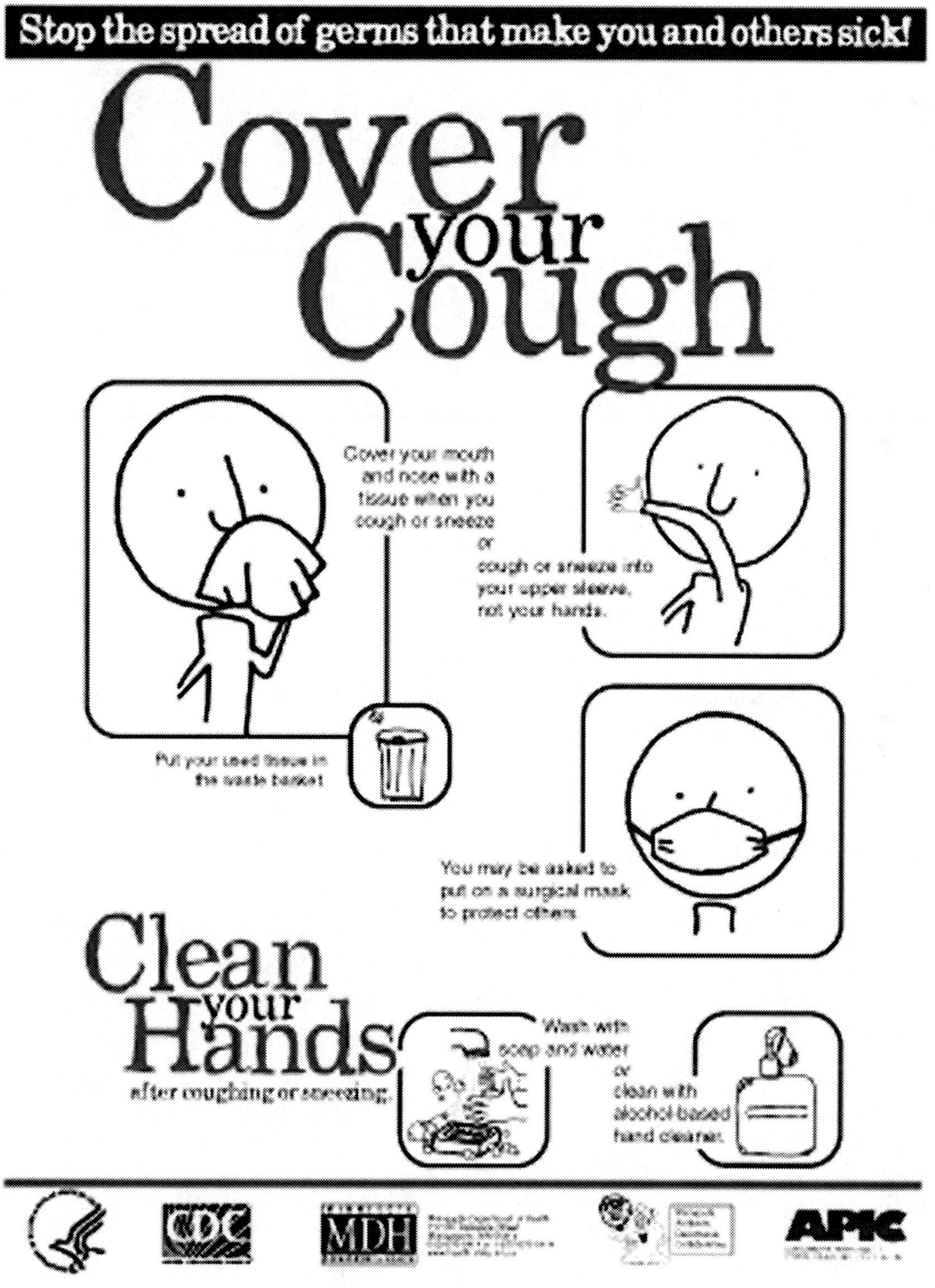

**Stop the spread of germs that make you and others sick!**

# Cover your Cough

Cover your mouth and nose with a tissue when you cough or sneeze

or

cough or sneeze into your upper sleeve, not your hands.

Put your used tissue in the waste basket.

You may be asked to put on a surgical mask to protect others.

# Clean your Hands

after coughing or sneezing.

Wash with soap and water

or

clean with alcohol-based hand cleaner.

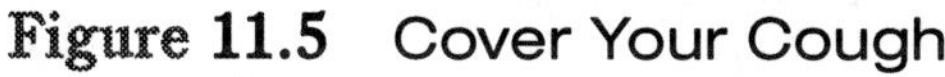


**Figure 11.5** Cover Your Cough

Source: www.cdc.gov/flu/protect/covercough.htm.

Table 11.2 Levels of Infection Control

| Control Level | Control Type | Effect | Procedure |
|---|---|---|---|
| Low | Sanitization | Removes contaminants | Cleaning with soap and detergents |
| Medium | Disinfection | Destroys many pathogens | Using chemical solutions |
| High | Sterilization | Destroys all microbes and spores | Using several different methods—see Figure 11.6 |

provides some helpful tips from the CDC about ways to keep germs from spreading. The CDC website has many helpful posters and flyers on a variety of health issues. Many are easy to download and all are free.

There are three levels of infection control, as shown in Table 11.2. The lowest level is **sanitization,** cleaning the surface using soap or detergent. This process will reduce the number of microbes. Warm, soapy water should be used to thoroughly clean surfaces.

**Disinfection** is the second level of infection control. Common disinfectants like bleach, when used properly, can destroy many pathogens and other microbes. Disinfectants are more effective if the items have been sanitized first.

The process that destroys all forms of microorganisms and bacterial spores is **sterilization.** As the highest level of infection control, sterilization is used on medical instruments. Any medical instrument that breaks the skin, contacts surgical incisions, or becomes contaminated during a procedure should be sterilized. There are five different methods of sterilization, as shown in Figure 11.6. Additionally, many medical offices use disposable sterile supplies that come in ready-to-use packages. These supplies are to be used once and discarded appropriately after use.

Not everyone in the medical office has the same exposure to infection under normal circumstances. Front desk staff members are less likely to be exposed to the same types of infections as clinical staff members. However, it is important for everyone to be aware of how germs and bugs are spread and to take the right precautions to avoid the spread of disease.

Autoclaving—high pressure/steam heat
Immersion in approved chemical solutions
Dry heat ovens if the instruments would be damaged by either steam or chemicals
Microwaving
Sterilization gases such as ethylene oxide (normally only in hospitals)

**Figure 11.6** Types of Sterilization

## Pandemics

In the past several years, we have heard much about the bird or avian flu, and the term *pandemic* has been used a lot. A **pandemic** is an epidemic that is spread over wide areas of the world and affects large numbers of people. The CDC says that a flu pandemic occurs when a new influenza virus emerges for which people have little or no immunity, and for which there is no vaccine. The disease spreads easily person-to-person, causes serious illness, and can sweep across the country and around the world in a very short time.

Despite all the publicity about the HFNI (bird) flu virus, it has not yet become a pandemic. Does that mean we will never see a pandemic again? Most experts believe that flu pandemics occur in cycles of 10 to 30 years. The last flu pandemic took place in 1969 (see Table 11.3). As you can see, the medical community was able to reduce the number of deaths from flu pandemics partly because it has a much better understanding of how a pandemic spreads. Therefore, we need to have both personal and office plans in place

**Table 11.3** Flu Pandemic Deaths

| Year | U.S. Deaths | Worldwide Deaths |
|---|---|---|
| 1918–1919 | 675,000+ | 50,000,000+ |
| 1957–1958 | 70,000+ | 1,000,000 to 2,000,000 |
| 1968–1969 | 34,000+ | 700,000+ |

Source: Centers for Disease Control and Prevention.

because it could happen again. Authorities worldwide are making plans, but because it has been so long since this country and the world have seen a true pandemic, we tend to dismiss the potential problems. Medical facilities should be particularly concerned, as the patients with the flu will be seeking care. According to the CDC, it is difficult to predict when the next influenza pandemic will occur or how severe it will be. Wherever and whenever a pandemic starts, everyone around the world is at risk. Countries might, through measures such as border closures and travel restrictions, delay arrival of the virus, but they cannot stop it.

The characteristics of a pandemic include the following:

- The disease will spread rapidly from person to person due to little or no immunity.
- Substantial numbers of people will require some form of medical care.
- Normal flu viruses have a major effect on older and younger individuals; a pandemic flu will impact all ages.
- Death rates are high.
- The health care systems are unable to manage the spread of the disease as there will not be enough staff, hospital beds, and equipment to manage a large influx of patients.
- The need for vaccine will outstrip the supply; the antiviral drugs needed in the early stages of the pandemic will be depleted quickly.
- Difficult decisions will have to be made about who gets the vaccines and antiviral medications.
- Past flu pandemics have come in two or three waves, each lasting six to eight weeks.
- Travel bans, school closures, and other restrictions will create problems.
- Caring for a sick family member and fear of exposure will create significant employee absenteeism.



Communication and information are critical components of pandemic response. The CDC has indicated that education and outreach are critical to preparing for a pandemic. Understanding what a pandemic is, what needs to be done at all levels to prepare for pandemic influenza, and what could happen during a pandemic helps us make informed decisions both as individuals at our practices and as a nation. Your practice needs a plan in place. This plan will help you deal with a pandemic or local flu epidemic that becomes crippling.

Experts agree that all medical offices should have a response plan in place for an epidemic and/or pandemic. The first step in establishing that plan is based on the practice type and location. Rural practices will have to prepare to be a major focal point for their community. Many times, options for inpatient care are limited in rural settings, and the medical communities will need to look at ways to create space for higher than normal levels of hospitalized patients. Urban and metropolitan practices have more resources at hand, but it will require significant coordination among the various area agencies.

States have emergency response plans in place. Usually they are coordinated through the local department of health. In all likelihood, the physicians in your practice are already aware of and may be participating in the necessary planning for an emergency. However, every practice must also look internally and plan for the emergency.

Although every practice's plan will differ, there are key components that all practices should identify for their internal plan. The CDC has a complete checklist of how to prepare for a pandemic on its website (www.pandemicflu.gov/plan/pdf/medofficesclinics.pdf). You can use this checklist to identify the strengths and weaknesses of your plan, or to start a plan.

The first step in the CDC checklist is to develop a structure for planning and decision making. This includes identifying members of a planning committee (if appropriate due to the size of the practice) as well as identifying point-of-contact people within the practice.

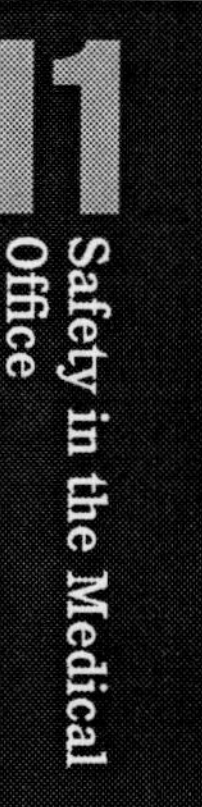


The second and third steps are to develop a written plan. The plan should include:

- Surveillance and detection of pandemic influenza in the population served.
- A communication plan within the practice and with key public health contacts, as well as health care entities.
- Education and training for all medical office staff.
- Informational materials for patients that are in language and reading level appropriate for the population being served. Many of these materials are available on the CDC website.
- A plan for triage and management of patients during the pandemic.
- An infection control plan.
- A vaccine and antiviral use plan.
- An occupational health plan that includes handling of staff who become ill, when personnel may return to work, when personnel who are symptomatic but well enough to work will be permitted to continue working, and personnel who need to care for their ill family members.
- Issues related to surge capacity—the influx of patients and staff and supply shortages.

Both the CDC and the individual states have a wealth of information available about emergency preparedness and response. The CDC contains information for both the public and the medical community on bioterrorism, chemical emergencies, mass casualties, natural disasters, and radiation emergencies. In Chapter 7, we covered preparing your electronic and other records for possible disaster. Hurricanes Katrina and Rita, as well as other natural disaster events, have made us all more aware of being better prepared for catastrophe. Much of the planning your practice does for a pandemic will also serve well in the event of other emergencies.

## Summary

Safety is everyone's responsibility. In the medical practice, not only do we have to be aware of the commonsense things like washing our hands and covering our mouths when we cough, but also those procedures that reduce the chances of anyone becoming infected. Constant attention to infection control should be a day-to-day activity.

The threat of pandemic or other major emergency affecting the community must be treated seriously. As a country, we are still learning much about how to react to these types of threats. In an emergency, common sense sometimes disappears, so well-prepared health and medical personnel is a must. Both the CDC and your local health department are valuable resources to help everyone prepare for the unthinkable.

# Chapter 12

# Managing Stress

## Introduction

*"I am so stressed out" is a common statement heard in offices and homes. What causes stress? Is there good and bad stress? How can I deal with the conflict in the office? I have a difficult boss, how can I learn to work with him? How can we communicate better with difficult patients? How should we work with patients to help them get well? How do I deal with the difficult fellow employee who manages to ruin a perfectly good day because of her attitude and smart remarks? All of these things and more cause us stress in the office. In this chapter we will look at what stress is, how to manage it in the workplace, and how to recognize our own stress levels. We will also look at stress reducers.*

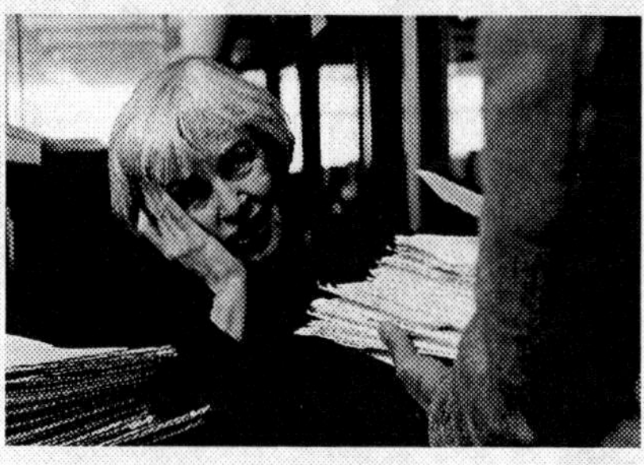

## Chapter Outline

## Stress Defined

Stress is tension. Our body's reaction to stress may include increased heart rate, tense muscles, increased blood pressure, and sweating. Stressed individuals may seem confused, irritable, or unable to concentrate. We sometimes have these symptoms even in situations that cause good stress, such as getting married or having a baby. Stress also can be caused by negative events such as divorce or death. In addition, certain stressful situations affect individuals differently. For example, a job interview can be stressful for one person but a challenge for another. Learning new computer software can be stressful for one individual but an opportunity for another.

### Common Misconceptions About Stress

There is a lot of talk about stress, and there are some common misconceptions that are important to understand. The first misconception is that we always know when we are under stress. Often we become so accustomed to stress that we are unaware of it. The second misconception about stress is that it affects only those individuals who live high-pressure lives. Stress may affect anyone at any level. You don't have to be in a high-level job to experience stress. Third, it is a misconception to believe that the only way to lower stress is to change your situation or take medication. Much of our stress is based on how we perceive the world, so if we change our perception, we may be able to change our stress levels. Related to that misconception is the idea that stress is caused by events that happen to us. It isn't the events in and of themselves; it is how we view the events. The last misconception is that our emotional reactions have a life of their own and cannot be controlled. We are able to change our behavior and our emotional reactions by changing how we think. Our world is stressful, but we are able to reduce our stress levels.

## Causes of Stress

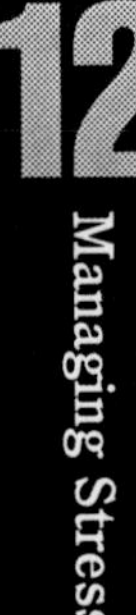


There are big stressors and little stressors. Big stressors are those life-changing events that we don't deal with every day. Figure 12.1 lists common big stressors. Little stressors are those day-to-day problems that usually affect us for only a short period. Figure 12.2 lists little stressors.

Big stressors may affect us for a long time, whereas little stressors are those daily annoyances that sometimes get out of control and lead to inappropriate behavior. Some stressors we can control; others are out of our control. Stress levels are different for everyone. Some people seem to take everything in stride and not get stressed, while others react to every little annoyance in life as if it were a major problem.

- Marriage
- Divorce
- Death of a family member or friend
- Illness
- Hospitalization—yours or family members
- Having a baby
- Changing jobs
- Changing your financial situation—good or bad
- Children leaving or coming back home
- Losing a job
- Retirement
- Sexual problems
- Personal success—a promotion or an award
- Moving
- Remodeling your home
- Problems at work where your job may be at risk
- Significant debt or overspending

**Figure 12.1** Big Stressors

- Traffic
- Weather
- Deadlines (which can become a big stressor if they are constant)
- Spouse and/or children running late
- Loud noises
- Rude people
- Long waiting lines
- Malfunctioning equipment
- People who are late
- People who talk too much
- Poor service at the store
- Misplaced items
- Office drama

**Figure 12.2** Little Stressors

## Stress at Work

The **National Institute for Occupational Safety and Health (NIOSH)** defines job stress as the harmful physical and emotional responses that occur when the requirements of the job do not match the capabilities, resources, or needs of the workers. It is important not to confuse job challenges with job stress. Challenges on the job motivate us, and when we meet the challenge, we feel satisfied. When people say "a little bit of stress is good for you," they are probably referring to the challenges of the job. But when the challenge turns into job demands that cannot be met, satisfaction may turn into stress. As an example, dealing with difficult patients is a challenge. Continuously not having enough staff to answer the phones and deal with the patients may cause job stress.

NIOSH reports that 40% of workers reported that their job was very or extremely stressful. Twenty-five percent of those surveyed thought their job was the number one stressor in their lives. As Americans, we are working longer and harder. It is often hard to distinguish when personal stress is adding to or may even be causing additional stress on the job. For example, if an employee is dealing with any of the stressors shown in Figure 12.1, the person may not perform well on the job or may react more strongly to those conditions on the job that normally are challenges, not stressors.

### Job Conditions That Lead to Stress

What are the major conditions that lead to stress in the workplace? The nature of the business of health care makes stress an everyday occurrence. Dealing with people who are sick is often difficult. Stress levels increase when the job conditions are such that it is impossible to do a good job all the time. Figure 12.3 outlines some examples of what conditions you might see in the medical office that may create high levels of stress. You probably can make your own list of conditions that apply in your office.

It is important to remember that continued bad stress affects our health. There is evidence to suggest that health care expenditures are nearly 50% greater for workers who report high levels of stress. Over the years, many studies have looked at the relationship between job stress and health. Early signs of stress include mood and sleep disturbances, upset stomach, and headaches as well as disturbed relationships with family and friends. These are all quick to develop and easy to recognize and to treat.

The long-term effects of job stress are harder to determine. Many chronic diseases take a long time to develop and may be influenced by other factors than stress. However, evidence is building that stress plays an important role in several types of chronic health problems. Psychological disorders, cardiovascular disease, and musculoskeletal disorders are the most common.

***The Design of the Tasks.*** Heavy workload, infrequent rest breaks, long work hours and shiftwork; hectic and routine tasks that have little inherent meaning do not utilize workers' skills, and provide little sense of control.

**Example:** Susan works at the front desk of the medical office and is expected to answer the phones and greet all patients for a three-physician general practice. She has no backup for the phones, so if a patient is at the front desk asking questions and the phones are ringing, there is little she can do to manage both tasks.

***Management Style.*** Lack of participation by workers in decision making, poor communication in the organization, lack of family-friendly policies.

**Example:** The practice manager is rude to her employees and rarely communicates changes to be made, but is upset when things go wrong, sometimes yelling at employees in front of patients.

***Interpersonal Relationships.*** Poor social environment and lack of support or help from coworkers and supervisors.

**Example:** Tony, the medical records clerk, is the youngest employee in the practice as well as the only male staff member. His fellow employees routinely exclude him from conversation and assume that because he is a male, he will do all the physical work (moving boxes, fixing things, etc.) that is necessary in the practice.

***Work Roles.*** Conflicting or uncertain job expectations, too much responsibility, "too many hats to wear."

**Example:** Theresa is the office coordinator. She is also the billing manager for the practice. The physicians tell her that getting the statements out is her primary responsibility, but they also expect her to help the office staff in answering the telephones and checking out patients.

***Career Concerns.*** Job insecurity and lack of opportunity for growth, advancement, or promotion; rapid changes for which workers are unprepared.

**Example:** The large group practice is switching to the electronic medical record. Little training has been provided to the support staff. In addition, the three medical records clerks are uncertain if they will retain their jobs. No one will offer them any information.

***Environmental Conditions.*** Unpleasant or dangerous physical conditions such as crowding, noise, air pollution, or ergonomic problems.

**Example:** Since medical practices are in offices, there are rarely dangerous physical conditions unless some safety hazards are present. Because medical office staff sit most of the time, having appropriate desk chairs may be a problem. Lighting conditions may also cause eye strain.

**Figure 12.3** Job Conditions That Lead to Stress

Source: National Institute for Occupational Safety and Health, *Stress . . . at Work*, DHHS (NIOSH) Publication No. 99-101.

Stressful working conditions as a part of the job can lead to lower productivity and lower profitability. NIOSH reports that stressful working conditions are associated with increased absenteeism, tardiness, and intentions by workers to quit. Additionally, some studies suggest that organizations that are considered "healthy organizations" have a better bottom line.

## What Is a Healthy Organization?

It is one that has low rates of illness, injury, and disability in its workers and is also competitive in the marketplace. Research done by NIOSH indicates that there are several organizational characteristics associated with healthy workplaces and high levels of productivity. Figure 12.4 lists those characteristics.

It is important to remember that everyone in the organization will have a slightly different viewpoint about the four characteristics shown in Figure 12.4. No organization is perfect. For example, you may see yourself as the hardest-working employee in the practice. You may be stressed because you don't believe you have been recognized for your performance. However, your definition of working hard and the organization's perception of hard work may differ. If others in the organization are being recognized for work performance and you aren't, you might want to reassess your definition of appropriate work performance. When everyone around you is getting promoted and you are not, you need to review your overall performance with your supervisor. You must also look at long-term performance. Improving your performance over just a few months probably won't result in a promotion or pay increase.

Many organizations possess several but not all of the characteristics of a healthy organization. In small offices, the opportunities for career development may be limited by the size of the organization. Small, healthy workplaces focus on recognizing performance and

- Recognition of employees for good work performance
- Opportunities for career development
- An organizational culture that values the individual worker
- Management actions that are consistent with organizational values

**Figure 12.4** Characteristics of a Healthy Workplace

Source: National Institute for Occupational Safety and Health, *Stress . . . at Work,* DHHS (NIOSH) Publication No. 99-101.

demonstrating how much they value the individual worker. In larger healthy organizations, you will see more opportunities for career development, but perhaps the larger organization may not always recognize employees for strong work performance.

Much of this is also about perception. What you see as recognition, opportunities, and management actions that support organizational values may differ from how others view these actions.

## What Should Organizations Do to Reduce Stress?

Because stress is different for each individual, organizations need to look at the total environment to ensure that everything possible is being done to reduce job stress in general. It is not possible to create a work environment without stress, but employers should take responsibility for preventing as much job-related stress as possible. Working toward reducing the stress in an organization may in and of itself cause some additional stress to begin with. Figure 12.5 lists ideas to help the organization change to help reduce job stress.

Getting an organization to seriously look at its stress problems is not easy. There are no standardized manuals that, if followed, will lead to stress reduction. Before implementing a major stress reduction program, it is important to determine if the stress may be resolved

Employers should:

- Make sure the workload is in line with employees' capabilities and resources.
- Design jobs to provide meaning, stimulation, and opportunities for employees to use their skills.
- Clearly define employees' roles and responsibilities.
- Give employees' opportunities to participate in decisions that affect their job.
- Improve communication—let employees know about possible career development and future employment prospects.
- Provide social interaction opportunities.
- Whenever possible, establish work schedules that are compatible with demands and responsibilities outside the job.

**Figure 12.5** Reducing Job Stress in the Organization

Source: National Institute for Occupational Safety and Health, *Stress . . . at Work,* DHHS (NIOSH) Publication No. 99-101.

by a simple solution. For example, if one workflow process is the source of stress, work toward fixing the workflow process. However, if the practice is experiencing low productivity, a high turnover of employees, absenteeism, and patient complaints, it is time to look at identifying the causes of the stress and possible solutions.

NIOSH suggests using a three-step approach, as shown in Figure 12.6, to help identify the problems. To be successful, every organization should first begin to build general awareness about the causes, costs, and control of job stress. Top management commitment is essential to any stress prevention program, and input should come from all employees. Employees should be involved in all phases of the program. If the stress is causing high levels of lost productivity, the organization should consider hiring a professional that is trained in stress reduction programs.

We spend a great deal of time at our workplace. We can't always have the perfect job, with little stress, so learning how to manage our stress is important for our overall success and well-being.

1. Identify the problem
   - Hold group discussions
   - Design and implement an employee survey
   - Measure employee perceptions of job conditions, stress, health, and satisfaction
   - Collect objective data
   - Analyze data to identify problem locations and stressful conditions
   - Attempt to keep the survey participants' answers anonymous
2. Design and implement change
   - Target the source of the stress
   - Propose and prioritize change strategies
   - Communicate planned changes to employees
   - Implement change
3. Evaluate the change
   - Conduct both short- and long-term evaluations
   - Measure employee perceptions of job conditions, stress, health, and satisfaction
   - Include objective measures
   - Refine the change strategy and return to step 1 if necessary

**Figure 12.6** Stress Prevention Plan for Organizations

Source: National Institute for Occupational Safety and Health, *Stress . . . at Work,* DHHS (NIOSH) Publication No. 99-101.

## Managing and Preventing Stress at the Personal Level

There is a difference between preventing stress and managing stress. Although we may say we would love a life free of stress, we would probably be very bored. A stress-free life probably means you are dead! However, there are some stressors we may be able to prevent or avoid. Other stressors are unavoidable and will require us to manage our response to the stressful situation.

At the beginning of the chapter, we identified the big and little stressors in life. Sometimes more than one big stressor is a part of our life, and often a lot of little stressors can become a big stressor for us. How do we know when we are so stressed that it may be affecting our health? How do we determine if we are able to prevent the stress or if we must manage it? First, let's look at the symptoms of stress.

### Stress Symptoms

Our body gives us some physical clues. Some of the physical warning signs include sweaty palms or body sweat (that is not due to warm air temperature), tense muscles, chronic tiredness, nervous stomach, headaches, heartburn, and weight gain or loss. Many of us are emotional eaters, and we either eat too much or not enough when we are stressed beyond normal limits.

Second, we react emotionally when we are stressed. We are irritable, sometimes confused, we become angry quicker, we can't concentrate, we can't sleep, we are always anxious, we worry about every little thing, and we may have frequent mood swings.

Last, there may be behavioral warning signs. We overreact to little things, we act on impulse, we change jobs frequently, we call in sick when we really aren't, and we might begin using drugs or alcohol. Some people begin to withdraw from others and feel agitated a lot.

To determine if your stress levels are possibly affecting your health, you need to first assess your current stressors. There are three categories: major life changes, ongoing problems, and accidental problems or hassles. Again, it is the big stressors and the little stressors. Most of the major life changes and ongoing problems are big stressors. The accidental problems and hassles are little stressors. Make a list of those events that cause stress in your life. The list will help you identify what you can change or eliminate and what you must accept. For those stressors that you must accept, you will need to determine how to cope with them.

Identify how you currently cope with stress. Are you using healthy or unhealthy coping techniques? For example, are you exercising (healthy) or are you drinking alcohol more frequently (unhealthy)? Are you procrastinating (unhealthy) or attempting to balance your work and personal life (healthy)? Are you taking breaks (healthy) or working through lunch (unhealthy)? Do you feel sorry for yourself (unhealthy) or are you using positive thoughts (healthy)? If you find that you are using more unhealthy techniques to reduce stress than healthy techniques, it is time for reassessment.

Stress is a highly personalized problem, so the resolutions are also highly personalized. Some people analyze the situation and take action to deal directly with the issues. Others are more emotionally oriented and prefer to talk it out or use other social supports to work through the stressful period. A third coping style is to use distractions to keep your mind off the situations that are causing the stress. All of us may use all of these styles, depending on the situation. The key is to remember that you will need to modify your behavior to reduce the stress levels.

## Preventing Stress

Some generalized techniques have been found to help prevent the physical, emotional, and behavioral reactions to stress. Figure 12.7 provides you with some of those techniques.

***Avoid*** controllable situations that cause stress. For example, instead of taking a break with an employee whose favorite activity is to gossip negatively about others in the office, change your break time.

***Exercise*** on a routine basis. Most experts suggest that at least 45 minutes of aerobic exercise four to five times a week are necessary to help maintain a healthy lifestyle. If we feel better, we are less likely to react to the little stressors.

***Eat right.*** As health care professionals, we all know that eating right makes a difference. We also know how hard it is to eat right. Balanced, nutritious meals and healthy snacks help us reduce our stress levels.

***Balance*** your life among work, family, and fun. There are times when our jobs take priority, but we should always leave time for family and fun.

***Sleep*** enough so that you start your day rested and ready. Continuous lack of sleep makes most people cranky and irritable.

***Set realistic goals*** for yourself. It may be that you need to just set some goals, but set goals that you can attain.

***Prioritize*** wherever you have control. Recognize that you can't do it all.

***Change*** some of the things you have control over. Recognize those things that you cannot control and learn to not get upset or worried.

**Figure 12.7** Stress Prevention Tips

Source: National Institute for Occupational Safety and Health, *Stress . . . at Work,* DHHS (NIOSH) Publication No. 99-101.

They won't always work, but these ideas will help prevent negative stress that may cause health problems. In some cases, avoiding stress is the best solution. However, we do not always have the luxury of avoiding the causes of stress. We must then work on how to manage the stress.

Limiting our caffeine and alcohol intake, as well as eating vitamin C–rich foods, proteins, and complex carbohydrates, will help in stress reduction. You will improve your health in general if you stay away from caffeine and sugar. Many people eat more when stressed, and often it is the kind of food that is not good for healthylifestyles.

There is little evidence that smoking reduces stress. Much of the research suggests that smokers are more stressed than nonsmokers, and some studies have shown that individuals report feeling less stressed after they have quit smoking. There is a lot of evidence that smoking is bad for us in general, so smoking is not a good choice for a variety of reasons.

## Managing Stress

So, how do we deal with stressful situations—those situations that we cannot make go away or reduce? Our ability to manage our stress so that we don't overreact on a continuous basis is important for a healthy lifestyle.

Figure 12.8 identifies some tips for managing stress. Recognize when you will have stress, and work on managing yourself in the stressful situation. When you are stressed at work, try to concentrate on the positive aspects of your job. Go into situations positively, rethinking your negative thoughts. For example, instead of thinking or saying "I will never get this done in time," think or say "I will be as prepared as I can be and get as much done as I can." Reducing stress requires that you believe in yourself. It also requires that you rethink how you view the situation. It requires that you begin to modify your behavior. You need to be aware of your physiological and emotional reactions to stress, as well as recognizing what you can change. It is important to use healthy coping skills all the time. Using them will help you be ready for the times when you are feeling overwhelmed.

How we perceive stressful events and how we react to them determine the impact on our health. If we always respond in a negative way to stress, we are likely to see our health and happiness suffer. We may also lose our job and our family relationships if we don't learn to deal with the stress. The reality is that attitude is everything when it comes to preventing and managing stress.

There is a fine line between feeling stressed out but functioning and being *burned out* and in need of professional help. The term *burnout* was first used in 1974 by Herbert Freudenberger. He described burnout as the "collapse, exhaustion or extreme fatigue

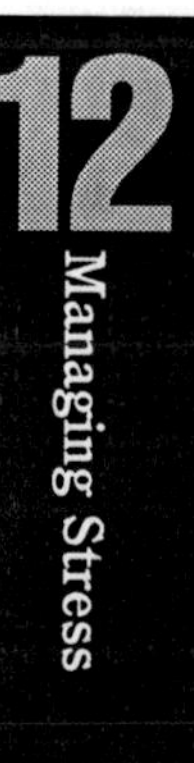

**Identify** sources of conflict and try to resolve them. If they aren't resolvable, work on ways to spend less time in the situation.

**Be realistic** about what you can and cannot do. Do not be afraid to admit that you may have overcommitted or that you simply cannot take on another responsibility.

**Get organized.** Look at the time wasters in your day—both at home and at work—and see how you can better organize the situation.

**Redirect excess energy.** Do volunteer work, clean out your closet, exercise more. Do something you like.

**Stay focused** When we are stressed, we often lose sight of the real problem.

**Learn** some relaxation techniques. Imagine yourself in a quiet place. Use relaxation techniques such as meditation or deep breathing. Figure out what works for you.

**Rely** on the support of family and friends. Don't be afraid to share your feelings at the appropriate time.

**Don't overreact** Ask yourself if it is really worth getting upset or worried about.

**Maintain a sense of humor** The old saying "laughter is the best medicine" was probably developed by someone with a lot a stress. Read the comics, go to a funny movie, or just relax with friends.

**Seek professional help** if your ability to manage the stress becomes consistently overwhelming. There are support groups as well as psychologists that may help you deal with the stress.

Figure 12.8 Managing Stress

resulting from an excessive demand of energy, strength or resources." **Burnout** is a psychological condition brought about by unrelieved stress that results in exhaustion, lower resistance to illness, increased pessimism, and possible depression. The important word in the definition is *unrelieved.* We all face stress, but when there is no relief from the sources of the stress, we may have burnout and need professional help.

How can we tell if we just have high stress levels or we are burned out? If we are asking the question, it is best to seek professional help. Some experts suggest that the symptoms of burnout may become so much a part of your life that you may think you have a physical problem and not recognize the psychological problem.

## Summary

*Stress* is a widely used term and is often misunderstood. There are misconceptions about stress and whether it is good or bad for us. A certain degree of stress probably is helpful in maintaining good mental and physical health. Organizations can learn to be proactive in preventing and managing stress. Individuals can reduce their stress levels by using a wide variety of techniques. The physical and mental well-being of the employees can contribute to a positive bottom line for the medical office. The key to reducing stress is to be ready to accept a possible change in your perceptions about the situation at hand. A positive attitude creates a stronger workplace and healthier lifestyle.

# Glossary

## A

**Account** Individual patient's record of charges and payment.

**Accounting** Overall financial information of the practice, including the management of its assets and liabilities.

**Accounts payable** Amount of money owed by the practice to vendors and employees.

**Accounts receivable** Total amount of money owed to the practice by the patients.

**Adjustment** Discounts applied to the total charge for services based on a contract with the third-party payer. Adjustments are not write-offs for bad debt.

**Americans with Disabilities Act (ADA)** Federal law requiring that all businesses ensure that people with disabilities have access to buildings and offices.

**Assets** Resources owned by the organization. Includes accounts receivable, furniture, and equipment—anything with an economic value related to the practice.

## B

**Balance** Difference between the debits and the credits.

**Beneficiary** Person or persons insured.

**Bookkeeping** Recording of the financial information, such as charges and payments.

**Burnout** Psychological condition brought about by unrelieved stress that results in exhaustion, lower resistance to illness, increased pessimism, and possible depression.

## C

**Capitation** Payment method where providers are reimbursed a fixed amount per member per month and must provide all care for that reimbursement.

**Centers for Disease Control and Prevention (CDC)** This federal agency's mission is to promote health and quality of life by preventing and controlling disease, injury, and disability.

**Centers for Medicare and Medicaid Services (CMS)** Agency of the U.S. Department of Health and Human Services that sets the rules for Medicare and Medicaid.

**Charity care** Care provided for free to patients who cannot pay. This is not the same thing as bad debt write-off.

**Civilian Health and Medical Program of the Department of Veterans Affairs (CHAMPVA)** Coverage for surviving family members of a veteran. Normally, CHAMPVA is available only when the veteran has a service-connected disability.

**CMS-1500** Approved form for completing a claim for payment for outpatient health care services rendered.

**Coinsurance** Balance owed by the patient after the insurance payments have been applied.

**Combining form** Word root where a vowel is added at the end of the word root to help make the term easier to pronounce.

**Confidentiality** Process in which medical records are maintained to avoid unapproved viewing of the information.

**Consent** Patient gives permission for the exams, tests, and other procedures.

**Consolidated Omnibus Budget Reconciliation Act (COBRA) of 1985** Allows an individual to continue employer-sponsored health insurance for a limited period of time after job loss.

**Consultation** In medical practice, this is where the first physician sends a patient to another physician, usually a specialist, for care for a specific problem. The first physician expects that the patient will be directed back once the treatment for the specific problem is completed.

**Copayment** Payment made by the patient at the time of service. This payment may or may not be applied to the coinsurance, depending on the health insurance plan.

**Covered entities** Organizations that HIPAA specifies must follow various privacy rules.

**Credit** Payment applied to a patient's account.

**Credit balance** Balance that reflects that the practice has received more money than it should have for the services rendered. This balance is either refunded to the patient or may be applied to future services.

**Current Procedural Terminology, Fourth Edition (CPT)** Describes the procedures and services performed by physicians and other health care providers in code format.

## D

**Day sheet** or **daily journal** Record of all patient charges and patient receipts for those charges for that day.

**Debit** Charge added to the patient's account.

**Debit balance** Balance that reflects that the patient still owes money for services rendered.

**Deductible** Out-of-pocket expenses the patient is expected to pay before health insurance coverage begins.

**Demographics** Statistical information necessary to maintain patients' general information ( i.e., address, date of birth, employer, etc.).

**Disinfection** Second level of cleaning for infection control by using specific agents like bleach.

**Downcoding** When a provider submits a lower level code for a service that should have been coded at a higher level.

**Durable medical equipment (DME)** Items such as crutches, ventilators, orthotics, and other generally used equipment.

## E

**Electronic medical record (EMR)** or **electronic health record (EHR)** Medical record stored in an electronic format, rather than on paper.

**Encounter form** Sometimes called a superbill, this is the form where the provider records the procedures done and the diagnosis for each patient. An encounter form is created for each visit, not each procedure.

**Exclusive provider organization (EPO)** More restrictive type of preferred provider organization.

**Explanation of benefits (EOB)** Notice sent to all patients explaining how reimbursement of health care services was determined.

## F

**Federal truth-in-lending law** Law that says that businesses must be truthful to their customers (patients) about the interest rates charged for unpaid balances.

**Feedback** Response from the receiver of information.

**Fee-for-service** Term used to describe when a provider is reimbursed based on the actual charges or a portion of those charges based on the indemnity plan held by the patient.

## G

**Group health plans** Health insurance coverage provided on a group rather than an individual basis.

## H

**Hardware** Comprehensive computer term that describes all the physical parts of a computer.

**Healthcare Common Procedure Coding System (HCPCS)** Used for coding services provided by practitioners. It includes CPT codes and also codes for a variety of supplies, drugs, and durable medical equipment.

**Health Insurance Portability and Accountability Act (HIPAA) of 1996** Major federal law that covers both privacy in health care and the individual's right to portability of health care coverage.

**Health maintenance organization (HMO)** Health care system that assumes both the financial risk associated with providing comprehensive medical services and the responsibility for delivering those services.

## I

**Infection control** Effort made to control the presence of harmful microorganisms.

**Intangible** Something is that not easy to define or measure.

**International Classification of Diseases, Ninth Edition (ICD-9)** Provides a list of diagnostic codes for use in billing for services.

**Interoperability** Ability of different information technology systems and software applications to communicate and to exchange data accurately, effectively, and consistently and to use information that has been exchanged.

## J

**Journal** Recording of the day's financial activities. There may be several different journals created in a day—one to record charges and payments for patients seen that day and one to record the payments received by mail or electronically.

## L

**Liabilities** Money owed by the practice to vendors and employees.

## M

**Managed care** General term referring to the concept of limiting choice on the part of the patient for care.

**Matrix** Arrangement of appointment times for each provider.

**Medicaid** Assistance program funded by federal and state governments for low-income citizens that covers some health care costs.

**Medical asepsis** Methods and practice designed to prevent the spread of disease.

**Medical practice act** State act that provides regulations for physicians and other providers.

**Medicare** Type of insurance sponsored by the federal government that covers citizens over 65 without regard to income.

**Medigap** Supplemental insurance offered by private insurance companies to cover the costs that Medicare does not cover.

**Message** Content of the information sent by the sender.

## N

**National Center for Health Statistics (NCHS)** Federal agency responsible for collecting and distributing a variety of health care information to the American people.

**National Institute for Occupational Safety and Health (NIOSH)** Federal agency responsible for conducting research and making recommendations for the prevention of work-related injury and illness.

## O

**Occupational Safety and Health Administration (OSHA)** Federal agency that works to prevent injuries and protect the health of the American worker.

## P

**Pandemic** Epidemic that occurs over wide areas of the world and affects large numbers of people.

**Paralinguistics** Technical term for vocal communication that is separate from actual language; our tone of voice, our pitch, our inflection, and our loudness.

**Practice management system (PMS)** Specific software designed to manage the day-to-day business functions of a medical office.

**Precertification** Determination by a third-party payer that a particular procedure is necessary and will be paid for by the third-party payer at an agreed amount.

**Preferred provider organization (PPO)** Type of insurance plan that provides coverage through a network of selected health care providers.

**Prefix** First part of a word.

**Protected health information (PHI)** Health information defined by HIPAA as covered by privacy rules.

**Proxemics** Study of the amount of space we need around us, our "comfort zone."

## R

**Received on account (ROA)** Payments received from insurance companies and patients after the date of service

**Receiver** Person who is receiving the information sent by the sender.

**Referral** Differs from a consultation; the first physician is handing off treatment to a second physician.

**Release of information (ROI)** Process of following the law in releasing medical information about a patient.

**Remittance voucher** or **remittance advice** Summary sent to care providers outlining the amount to be paid and explaining why other amounts may not be paid.

**Reservoir host** Animal, human, or insect on which microorganisms live and grow.

## S

**Sanitization** Cleaning with soap or detergent.

**Sender** Person who is sending information.

**Software** General term that describes all of the instructions that are in computer programs.

**State Children's Health Insurance (SCHIP)** Funded by both the state and federal government, this insurance plan covers uninsured children whose families earn a certain amount.

**Sterilization** Highest level of infection control where all microorganisms and bacteria are destroyed.

**Suffix** Last part of a word.

**Superbill** See *Encounter form.*

## T

**Tangible** Something that is capable of precise identification or value.

**Third-party payers** Organization, usually an insurance company, that agrees to carry the risk of paying for health care services for a patient.

**Trial balance/daily edit report** Report created each day to determine if all charges and payments for services rendered that day have been entered properly and all cash and its equivalent accounted for.

**TRICARE** Insurance that covers both active-duty and retired members of the uniformed services.

## U

**Upcoding** When a provider submits a higher level code of service than was actually provided to obtain a higher reimbursement.

**U.S. Department of Health and Human Services Office for Civil Rights** Federal agency responsible for reviewing HIPAA violation complaints.

**Usual, customary and reasonable (UCR)** Insurance companies' determination of what is an acceptable charge in the fee-for-service process.

## W

**Word root** Part of the word that refers to the anatomy.

**Workers' compensation** Health care costs for an injury or illness related to a person's job are covered by workers' compensation.

**Write-off** Amount not expected to be paid because of bad debt. Often confused with adjustments, write-offs are only for money you thought you were going to receive, but don't because the patient doesn't pay. An adjustment is a recognition of a contractual agreement to accept less. Charity care is also an adjustment, but you have agreed not to charge the patient.

# Credits

Page **xii:** © Stockbyte/Punchstock; **4:** © Chronis Jons/Getty Images; **6:** © Larry Mulvehill/Corbis RF; **12:** © Getty Images/RF; **22:** © Jose Luiz Pelaez, Inc./Blend Images/Corbis RF; **28:** © McGraw-Hill Higher Education; **46:** © The McGraw-Hill Companies, Inc./Rick Brady, photographer; **53:** © Getty Images/RF; **60:** © The McGraw-Hill Companies, Inc./ Rick Brady, photographer; **78:** © McGraw-Hill Higher Education; **105:** © Dynamic Graphics/Jupiter Images RF; **121:** © Corbis/RF; **156:** © Getty Images/RF; **180:** © Corbis/RF; **195:** © Getty Images/RF.

# Index